A Sleep Divorce
How to sleep apart, not fall apart

A SLEEP DIVORCE

How to sleep apart, not fall apart

Jennifer Adams

Neil Stanley PhD

T

Troubador Publishing Ltd
Unit E2 Airfield Business Park
Harrison Road, Market Harborough
Leicestershire LE16 7UL
Tel: 0116 279 2299
Email: books@troubador.co.uk
Web: www.troubador.co.uk

ISBN 978 1 80514 256 0

British Library Cataloguing in Publication Data.
A catalogue record for this book is available from the British Library.

Printed and bound in Great Britain by 4edge Limited
Typeset in 10pt Helvetica Neue by Troubador Publishing Ltd, Leicester, UK

Dedicated to all couples who value and seek
a good night's sleep.

Contents

How To Get the Most Out of This Book

We both believe that understanding the social history and evolution of sleep, and the science of sleep, are useful to help you make sense of current sleep issues you are facing. (We assume that because you bought this book, there are some issues you are trying to resolve.)

However, we also understand that you may have bought this book to simply get some practical advice about separate sleeping. So, here's some guidance about how to navigate the pages ahead so you can get the most out what we have researched, learned, experienced, and now share with you.

Interested in the social history and influences on sleep?

Chapters 1 and 3, will give you insights into humans' social behaviour when it comes to sleep and bed sharing.

These chapters will take you through the history of human relationship with sleep, and the evolution of 'where we sleep and why'. Because of how important it is to us as humans, scholars and historians have been writing about sleep and beds for a long time, which informs a lot of our current bedtime practices. We also provide information for you about what the current thoughts about sleep and bed-sharing are.

Interested in the science of sleep?

Chapter 2 and appendix 1 are for you. Understanding the biology and physiology of why and how we sleep helps us understand our own body and why it does so many weird and wonderful things. Ever heard people talk about being a 'lark' or an 'owl' and wondered what on earth they are talking about? Ever thought a circadian rhythm was something at a South American dance concert? Well – Chapter 2 will tell you all you need to know about why your body is doing what it does when it comes to sleep.

Interested in how separate sleeping might work for you?

Head to Chapters 4, 5, 6 and 7. These chapters will take you through a process to determine if separate sleeping is for you, give you advice about how you can make it work, and offer suggestions about how you can respond to social perceptions and judgements about the practice. We offer a range of perspectives and solutions for couples who maybe just want to try sleeping differently, right through to making separate bedrooms work for you and talking confidently and comfortably about your choices.

Setting the Scene

This book came about when we were each invited to take part in a panel interview about separate sleeping for *HuffPost Live* (the online network of *The Huffington Post*). When the interview ended, we continued to talk about our shared interest in separate sleeping.

The initial reason Jennifer wanted to write about the issue of separate sleeping came from discussions had when revealed to others that she and her husband didn't share a bedroom (had never really shared one actually). Through these early discussions, Jennifer developed an interest in people's perceptions of separate sleeping. Her curiosity set her off on a mission to discuss the topic whenever the opportunity presented itself. What she found was an assortment of attitudes and honesty about the issue, and a recurring theme of reluctance to be open about the practice for fear of social judgement. While Jennifer had no concerns about sharing this aspect of her life (think 'heart' and 'sleeve' and you have her) she found there were many people who had similar arrangements, but different approaches to sharing them. Intrigued as to why people were so secretive about, what was for her and me, a practical solution to the problem of not being able to sleep at night because of sleeping incompatibilities her investigations began.

As a result of many conversations and the encouragement Jennifer received to share thoughts and opinions on separate sleeping, Jennifer published her work in *Sleeping Apart not Falling Apart* (Finch Publishing 2013),[1] which provides the bedrock upon which this book is built. She thought then, and still thinks now, there are many couples, or individuals in couples, who would like to know there are others who need sleep so badly that they prioritise it over and above the need to lie next to their partners at night. Jennifer thinks that they would like to know other couples sleep some nights or every night separately because of this need for quality sleep. And importantly, she thinks that knowing they are not alone in choosing to sleep separately would help them feel that their decision to do so is not that unusual.

Neil is a sleep expert and has been interested in the topic of separate sleeping for many years and has invariably practised what he preaches. His knowledge and research into couple's sleep provide the scientific underpinnings to Jennifer's interviews. Together we have written this book, with a purpose to provide information and practical suggestions for couples who struggle to sleep together. The book offers insights for couples who are curious to find out if there are options to solve their sleeping issues and who want to know how other couples are dealing with the problem. It may also prove useful to couples who are struggling to make sleeping separately work by providing a framework for them to review how they manage their current sleeping arrangements.

It is important to say up front that both of us support the many couples who sleep in the same bed night after night, snuggling together into blissful slumber, waking happily next to each other ready to face the day. We certainly don't think that sleeping apart is for every couple; just as we don't believe sleeping together is for everyone.

We also recognise that sleeping separately (especially in a separate room) is not an option readily available to everyone. Limited space, or certain domestic arrangements, may restrict the opportunity for one person to enjoy sleeping separately every night.

Where and how you sleep is only one aspect of a relationship and should assume an amount of importance that is right for each couple. As with every decision made in a partnership, all priorities need to be considered as part of a bigger picture. This includes respecting the other partner's needs as well as the needs of others in the equation such as children or extended family.

Jennifer had many, many conversations with people that she knew well and not so well. She also interviewed couples and individuals about their sleeping behaviours, both those who loved sleeping together and those who headed for separate rooms every night. Feedback from two articles she had published on Mia Freedman's *Mamamia* website and several radio interviews that followed gave her a wealth of feedback and comments on which to draw. All the formal and informal information gathered from these sources appears in different guises.

All names of people interviewed for the book or who submitted stories have had their names changed to respect their privacy. However, to give context to each story, the age of the person (as a minimum), and in most cases, their occupation, and the amount of time they have been with a partner has been included.

We are grateful to the many people who shared personal details and their stories. It is in the sharing of the personal that we gain an insight into who we are as people, and how we connect with all those around us – sometimes in the most unexpected and surprisingly honest and candid.

Jennifer's Bedtime Story

After marrying mid-2007, several people enquired as to how married life 'was treating me'. I could happily reply each time that 'all was well'. As my husband had moved into my house, those who knew me well enough would sometimes progress to asking how we were settling into a bedroom together. This was an easy answer.

No settling in required. We had separate bedrooms.

A common concern raised was that my marriage was either in some serious and early trouble or that my husband Fraser and I must be going through some growing pains and sleeping apart while we worked these issues through. I knew my marriage wasn't on shaky ground at all and would always reassure the person enquiring that all was well.

But back to the beginning – this is how I found myself as a dedicated separate sleeper.

In my early twenties and through to the mid-thirties, I had boyfriends with whom I very happily shared a bed. In fact, sharing a bed with a partner and snuggling into him to fall asleep was the fantasy I had read about in many a *Cleo* or *Cosmopolitan* magazine. I thoroughly enjoyed living out this fantasy at that stage of my life. I loved sleeping with my partners; the closeness of sharing a bed each night and the sharing of a space in a house or apartment that was ours. I didn't imagine this would ever change.

A two-year relationship at the age of 34 saw me sharing a bed with a new boyfriend. However, after about six months, I started to have issues with disturbed sleep. Not only did the boyfriend's snoring bother me, but he liked the room very cold every night.

As the relationship progressed, our disparate sleep needs created more and more tension in the relationship, and I became so stressed by his snoring and being so cold, that I spent three nights without any sleep, ironically caused by the stress of not sleeping. The situation became so dire that I was prescribed sleeping tablets. This was a low point as I began to ponder a future of either sleepless nights or repeat prescriptions.

(I do realise that there are people, such as mothers of young babies, who may think that three nights of sleeplessness is a bit lightweight and not much about which to complain. I have always admired those who can exist on little sleep, but my body's wiring is different, and I struggle without it.)

Faced with an ongoing dilemma, I started to sneak out to the spare room. However, the boyfriend did not approve and saw this strategy as an unnecessary overreaction. His solution was that I should sleep with earplugs every night. His interpretation of a traditional relationship involved sharing a bed every night – even if it meant that my comfort, much-needed nightly rest and health were suffering. My attempts to talk about the issue were met with much tongue clicking and dismissive annoyance and comments that 'lots of women deal with a snoring partner' so really... I should just get over it.

As it happened, I couldn't 'just get over it'.

A combination of factors (including the sleep issues) brought about the demise of the relationship. The ending, while sad, was also tinged with joy at the prospect of being free from the nightly trauma of sharing a bed with him. I returned to live in my house and oh so happily began sleeping in my own bed again. The freedom of choosing when and under what conditions I slept had never felt so welcome and important.

Then I met my husband. The throes of an early relationship mask many practical ills and incompatibilities. The first nights Fraser and I spent in a bed together were filled with the activities of a new relationship – dinners out, a healthy amount of alcohol and the enthusiastic passion a couple enjoys. This combination would work well to help us sleep through the night.

Once we started to settle down into the comfortable rhythm of who was going to stay at whose place, I started to experience restless sleep again. When we slept over at each other's homes, and I couldn't sleep, I would sneak to the couch if we were at my house, or the floor of the lounge at his place. This was not an ideal solution and did result in a less than satisfactory night's sleep and a little stress. However, as we weren't living together, the broken sleep was interspersed with regular, good sleep alone at my house.

An added complication is that Fraser rises at 5 am most mornings, and after a day's work prefers to be in bed by about 9 pm – at the latest! He did very well to stay up later when we first started seeing each other, but not surprisingly, he could not sustain the late nights.

After about four months, Fraser and I decided that

he should move into my house. The idea of sharing a bed was causing us both some consternation, but we didn't have an honest conversation about this aspect of sharing a home. The standard practice is quite simple; when you move in with someone, you share a bed with them. So that's what we did. Fraser moved in, and we started sharing a bed. We lasted a week.

Fraser's snoring kept me awake, and we didn't naturally 'fit' in the bed together – if that makes sense? As we were both in our late thirties, our ability to adapt to new situations was a skill deserting us both, so the situation wasn't one that either of us could easily overlook. Not that we confessed this to one another immediately. However, we did eventually have a chat.

During the chat, we agreed only to share a bed on the weekends as we needed to get our sleep during the week. That plan lasted about two weekends. A complicating factor for us was Fraser's snoring is not what I would describe as 'run-of-the-mill snoring', and in time we would find out that Fraser had sleep apnoea.

So, after three weeks of Fraser living in my house, we moved to sleeping in separate beds every night, and we were both happy with this arrangement. We still enjoyed lying in each other's beds before we went to sleep or upon waking, having a kiss goodnight and a kiss good morning, and dozing with each other in one bed, or the other, on the weekend.

This was how our set of rules evolved to manage the tyranny of separate rooms and the need to show each other that we were committed to the relationship.

On a very practical level, it became evident over time that sharing a room would have been problematic.

Fraser rises early most days and retires to bed early in the evening. In contrast, I am a night person. I will often stay up until 11.00 pm and beyond, and I do so love a lie-in on weekends. I am overly attached to reading in bed, and doing this in a shared bed when your partner is already asleep is awkward and inviting trouble.

There would also have been issues with room temperature and bed coverings. All added to a mounting list of bed incompatibilities and a realisation that separate rooms really were the best option for us. We both agreed that being resentful towards the other person because one of us had to give up the when and how of sleeping, wouldn't have made for a healthy relationship. Coming to this realisation made us feel more confident in the decision to sleep separately.

I know that our decision is not for everyone. Many people I know wouldn't dream of not sharing a bed every night with their partner; they see a shared bed as a cornerstone of their relationship. I believe our decision to sleep apart has strengthened our relationship. Because we spend every night apart, we are forced to be very honest with each other about our commitment to the relationship.

We take great care not to exclude each other from the part of our lives associated with a bedroom, as silly as that sounds. Lying around on each other's bed is commonplace, and neither room is considered a private space that the other can't enter.

We have been together for almost twenty years now, are very happy (notwithstanding the standard ups and downs any couple faces) and have a normal, functioning relationship. I often wonder if sleeping separately impacts on our relationship because we don't share the closeness of being in a bed together every night. When I weigh everything up though, I wonder if we would still be together had it not been for our decision to have separate bedrooms. I guess we will never know. Of most importance is that our sleeping arrangements work for us, and we are the only people who really understand why and how it works.

As humans, we tend to judge based on our own values and norms, and this is why we condemn or criticise others who are different. Because their decision is not one that we would make, we often don't attempt to understand it.

So, my sleeping story is not everyone's sleeping story. But I do know that there are thousands of couples whose sleeping story is similar to mine, and many thousands more who would like to at least try the storyline for themselves.

Neil's Bedtime Story (or how I became the 'separate sleeping' evangelist)

As a sleep researcher, you would expect that I am obsessed with getting a good night's sleep and indeed I try and do all that I can to ensure that I, and those that I am 'close' to, get good sleep. During my first serious long-term relationship, I bought a house with my partner, moved in together, and initially started sleeping in the same bed. However, my job as a sleep researcher meant that I was working odd hours and would often be getting up or going to bed at all times of the day or night.

Over time it became easier to sleep in separate beds to avoid disturbing each other occasionally, and over time, we realised that we slept better when we were apart. So separate sleeping became the norm. Our love life was perfectly normal; we just didn't sleep together. Now you could claim that sleeping separately contributed to our break-up, as she went to work in Switzerland and we just drifted apart.

When I started going out with the woman who was to become my, now ex-, wife, we slept separately from the start of our co-habiting. So far from being a portent to the end of our ten-year marriage, it was the real situation pretty much from the start of our relationship. During our marriage, we kept trying to sleep together in the same bed and even bought a 6ft bed and separate duvets in an attempt to find a solution, but we could never manage it for more than a couple of nights. It wasn't that either of us was a snorer or that anything particularly was the problem; it was just the presence of a tossing and turning person beside us that disturbed our sleep.

I don't remember us having any profound conversation about us sleeping separately; it was just a mature, pragmatic solution to a problem. We often discuss trying to sleep together, but it never worked. The important thing was that my wife in each of the houses we lived in together had her bedroom decorated and furnished according to her tastes, and I had mine. It wasn't that either of us was sleeping in the backroom, the guest room or the spare room.

When we went on holiday, we always tried to book a room with twin beds and if that was not available I, more often than not, slept on the floor. We divorced a couple of years ago, but I can categorically say that even if we had slept together during some or all of our relationship, this would have had made no difference to our decision to divorce.

In 2005 I co-authored one of the first papers objectively looking at couples sleep with my good friends in the Sociology Department of the University of Surrey – Meadows R, Venn S, Hislop J, Stanley N, Arber S. (2005) *Investigating couples' sleep: an evaluation of actigraphic analysis techniques*. Journal of Sleep Research 14 377-386[2] and this was followed up in 2009 with the publication of Meadows R, Arber S, Venn S, Hislop J, Stanley N. (2009) *Exploring the interdependence of couples' rest-wake cycles: an actigraphic study*. Chronobiology International 26(1) 80-92. I am one of the most quoted UK sleep experts in the media and as early as 2006,[3] I was quoted talking about sleeping together. But the media interest was really sparked after, the publication of the 2009 paper and my talk at the British Science Festival that year.[4]

But however much I endorsed the idea of separate beds/bedrooms I was never able to admit publicly that my wife and I slept apart because my wife did not want her elderly parents to find out.

Then one day when talking to a journalist from *The Sunday Times* I very much 'off the record' mentioned that I did sleep separately from my wife, but there was no way this could ever appear in public. Well, you can imagine my surprise when a couple of Sundays later, my wife was reading *The Sunday Times* Style magazine, and there was the statement that we slept separately. The genie was out of the bottle, so there was little point in future interviews not admitting to the fact that we slept apart. Thus, I became, almost by default, the 'separate sleeping' evangelist.

Sleep experts are very good at telling people what to do but rarely tell you what they themselves do. However, I am honest about my own sleeping arrangements so you can see that, to a large extent, I practice what I preach (feel free to browse my website www.thesleepconsultancy. com for further details). But in the spirit of honesty, I have to admit that the situation now is that I am in a new relationship, and I do often share a bed with my partner. There are a number of reasons for this.

We are in the first flush of the relationship.

We do not have the space for a separate bedroom.

She, as the English say 'sleeps like a log', (the Danish have in my opinion a much better phrase 'sleep like a shot cow') and so doesn't disturb me too much or encroach into my 'space'.

So, can indeed can 'love conquer all'? Perhaps, but do I sometimes dream about separate beds/bedrooms, or some nights wish there was another bed to which I could relocate? Of course, I do.

Important Note

Neither of us is medically qualified, so we must stress that if you are in any way worried by the problems you are having with your sleep or if you have medical problems that disturb your sleep you should always see a doctor as only they, in the full knowledge of your medical history, can recommend appropriate treatments.

ONE

A Social History of Sleep

"All this fuss about sleeping together.
For physical pleasure I'd sooner go to my dentist any day".

Evelyn Waugh[5]

Sharing a bed with a partner is one of the cornerstones of a relationship. Or at least that's the message of contemporary Western culture. In the last few decades, our cultural practices seem to equate a successful relationship with successfully sharing a bed. It's interesting logic. Recent research[6] has found that social dictates as to how a person should sleep can easily result in a discrepancy between cultural sleep norms and an individual's biological needs, and that sleep customs may not always be in the health interests of the individual.

But still, we keep jumping into bed with each other.

Socially accepted norms

A natural but complicated process, sleep is a fundamental human need that, like the need to eat, has a social lens of judgement cast over it. This lens ascribes so much more to sleeping than its basic physiological function. While there is no judgement over the act of sleeping itself, when two people commit to a personal relationship, there is an expectation that the couple will share a bed together each night to sleep. And while more couples than not are happy to walk this traditional path, why is sleeping apart so often frowned upon for couples? Why do so many people hide the fact that the ideal sleeping partner is themself? But most importantly, why do so many people endure sleepless night after sleepless night to just to conform to a social norm?

Sleeping, in itself, is an inherently selfish act you cannot share your sleep with anyone. Ironically many people choose to lie next to another person to do it. Gerhard Klösch, author of *Sleeping Better Together*[7] notes that "sleep, as well as being a process, is also a behaviour evidenced by rituals associated with its onset and end". And as we humans are wont to do, we like to share our behaviours and rituals with others. It's more fun that way.

Paul Rosenblatt, professor of family social science at the University of Minnesota and author of *Two in a Bed: The Social System of Couple Bed Sharing,*[8] writes about couples needing to learn to share a bed. Unfortunately, just as we can't all learn the mysteries of quantum physics, not everyone can learn to endure night after night of minimal or broken sleep simply for the sake of sharing a bed with the person they love – no matter how much fun those behaviours and rituals are.

Australian relationship expert and psychologist Jacqueline Saad says of sleeping apart, "We find the idea strange as society has conditioned us to expect that a couple must share a bed. It signifies the sharing and joining of personal and spiritual space. There is a stigma attached to sleeping in separate beds which traditionally implies a breakdown in the relationship."[9]

Stephanie Coontz, a professor of history and family studies at Evergreen State College in Washington State, argues that the weight of expectation on the marital bed is artificial and relatively new. She says,[10] "It represents this cookie-cutter model that developed in the early 20th century that told people you had to get every single need met by this constant togetherness. It doesn't tie in with what we know about the variety of coupled relationships that have worked in history." What's more, Coontz points out that the model doesn't fit contemporary life, in which couples marry later, bringing more experiences and habits to their relationships.

Writing in *Quartz* (2019)[11] Rosie Spinks noted: "Somehow, we have internalized the idea that to be in love is to put up with your partner's snoring, insomnia, or thrashing midnight movements until the day one of you dies – or you break up because you're so sleep-deprived." Is this what we truly seek from a loving relationship? Or is the 'ideal' relationship that is portrayed to us unattainable, and we have lost our ability to separate fact from fiction? And for the sake of an imagined perfection (or expectation), we can't be honest and admit that an aspect of a great relationship just doesn't work, and we need to find an alternative solution.

Esther Perel, a psychotherapist and relationship advisor, often speaks of the pressure couples put on each other by expecting that their partner will provide everything for them, be everyone for them, and provide all their needs – physically, emotionally, and mentally. Popular media has a lot to answer for in this space as it espouses romantic, never-ending love as the ideal. Perel notes that[12] "today, we turn to one person to provide what an entire village once did: a sense of grounding, meaning, and continuity". Boldly, I suggest that extrapolates to expecting our partner to be our ideal bed mate too!

Later in the book, we consider the history of shared sleeping, where, if your romantic/sexual partner was a horrendous snorer, it didn't matter. You could simply find another person in the shared sleeping space to sleep next to – after you had sex with your romantic partner. That was your choice when living in 'a village'. Now, once we choose someone to partner with – that's it! We think they are going to meet all our needs, every day, every night, every year… until they don't anymore, and we feel a bit hard done by. If you stop and reflect on the notion that one person is going to be perfect in every way, it is a bit of a big ask and an expectation that is rather doomed for failure.

The public face of sleep

As a culture heavily influenced by what we see in print and visual media, the portrayal of a couple sleeping

4

'together' has evolved from not showing couples together in bed at all, to the ubiquitous image of a married couple retiring to their twin beds (often clothed neck to ankle in flannelette) in many television shows and movies of the 1950s and 1960s, and finally to the point where couples, both hetero– and homosexual, are shown in a vast range of domestic arrangements, hopping into a bed together, without anyone raising an eyebrow.

Apparently one of the ultimate TV trivia questions is: who was the first couple to be shown on television sleeping in the same bed?[13] And it has different answers – depending on your definition of 'sleeping in the same bed'. According to most television trivia sources, *The Flintstones* (1960-1966) holds the distinction of being the first television program to show a couple in bed together – albeit an animated couple. Other trivia buffs[14] claim it was in a fifteen-minute program titled *Mary Kay and Johnny*, first screened in America in 1947. Actors Mary Kay and Johnny Stearns starred in a television-based domestic comedy as a real-life couple living in a Greenwich Village apartment, and to keep production costs down, the show was filmed in the couple's real apartment, with their real bed. However, there is contention as to whether Mary and Johnny were actually shown in the bed together, rather than just showing their bedroom with just one bed, leading viewers to the conclusion that they both slept there.

Another more popular show that featured a couple in bed was *I Love Lucy* in 1951. Two episodes in the first year showed Lucy (Lucille Ball) and Ricky (Desi Arnez) in what appeared to be a king-size bed. But when they crawled under the sheets, and under their separate blankets, it was apparent there were two beds pushed together, each one made up separately. So technically they weren't in the same bed. In later episodes, once little Ricky was born, the beds were separated by a nightstand. CBS suggested that the beds be pushed apart to diminish the impact of the suggested sexual history of Lucy and Ricky. Goodness knows how the viewers thought the child was conceived![15]

Indeed, whoever the first couple was, it is perhaps the pervasive image of domestic success involving a couple happily hopping into a bed every night and appearing rested and just as happy on waking the next morning that has helped to create the sought after image of night-time harmony to which we aspire. If you aren't blissfully slumbering next to your loved one as they do on TV and in the movies, does that mean there's something wrong?

I suppose you see it on TV. For me, it started with Bewitched. The happy couple sleeps together, and that's equated with marital bliss.
Suzette, 40, Administrative Assistant, married 17 years

Most couples on TV and in the movies always seem to get through a night's sleep without too much bother. They don't seem to be too troubled by their partner and often wake up with perfect hair and make-up. Maybe I'm generalising, but it isn't that way in my bedroom. Maybe I'm the one with the problem?
Lulu, 42, Legal Professional, married 6 years

But just as evolution continues on all fronts – we're

challenged by constant social change whether we like it or not – the dynamics of the traditional relationship model are open to reinvention. Pamela J. Smock, a University of Michigan sociologist, says, "Couples today are writing their own script, rewriting how to have a marriage."[16] She notes, though, that husbands are less willing to change familiar patterns. "Men are supposed to be one, dominant, and two, sexual," she says. "Their wives might be thrilled to have their own bedrooms and see it as a romantic thing—going back to romance, going back to dating, to intimacy—but the husband might not see it that way. As a social pattern, this could increase. A lot of people I know fantasise about living in the same apartment building as their husband—but in a separate apartment. That could be next."

I think it's a male ego thing that he wants me there. That's what it should be like and what we should do – according to him.
Kaye, 66, married 14 years

I know of males who insist that their wives sleep with them as they are the boss and are the dominant ones in the relationship. They think they have the right to say how things will be in their house.
Matt, 47, Senior Manager, married 20 years

A cultural shift in which more couples choose to sleep separately is reflected in statistics coming out of America. A survey by the National Sleep Foundation in 2001 found that 12% of married Americans were sleeping alone; by 2005, this figure had grown to 23%.[17] Studies in England[18] have found similar results with research in 2007 showing that more than a third of British couples frequently sleeping in separate rooms and a 2013 study by Ryerson University in Toronto suggest that between 30% and 40% of couples worldwide sleep apart.[19] In 2009 *The New York Times* cited a survey of builders and architects which predicted that by 2015, 60% of custom-built houses would have two master bedrooms. Gopal Ahluwalia, of America's National Association of Home Builders,[20] observed that this was a "market-driven demand that's going to continue".

> *...my husband snores and thrashes about, likes to sleep cold and throws all the covers over me, and wakes up at odd hours... mostly WAY earlier than I consider civilised. We retire in five years, to a house we're building. There will be TWO bedrooms equipped with king-sized beds for us, thanks.*
> MessyONE, www.slate.com

These statistics are not surprising when considered against the backdrop of cultural shifts coming out of social movements that gave women a louder voice and focused on equality in male/female relationships. The traditional role of woman as homemaker and carer of the husband is no longer a given. All the stereotypes of a woman as a wife—including those in the bedroom—have been substantially challenged in the last couple of decades.

> *This has never seemed to be a problem for us as we share both things. Chris baths the kids and does the vacuuming and still works pretty hard, and I do too.*

Since we have three children, it's not a big thing for us to sleep in separate beds, separate rooms – it's just not a big issue.
Liz, 41, Accountant, married for 10 years

A 2020 American study by *Sleep Standards*[21] found that 75% of participants believe that sharing sleep space results in poorer sleep quality, and close to 60% agree that sleeping separately would improve their sleep quality – to be fair, this was during COVID-19. Only 35% stated they would be ready to take the leap to separate sleeping long-term, which reflects a consistent response of between 30-40% of couples seeking separate sleeping arrangements.

When did sleeping together become the norm?

Looking back on the sleeping habits of our predecessors, a couple sleeping in the same bed every night has not always been the norm. It is a modern construct and hasn't always been the 'cool thing to do'.

Cultural, historical influences have always played a part in determining contemporary social behaviours. Where and with whom you sleep is one of those behaviours. Klösch tells us that "sleeping either in groups or in individual beds was the more common practice that researchers describe in humans from prehistoric societies to many contemporary non-European cultures" and that sleeping together is a "sociocultural phenomenon, a fashion, and a lifestyle".[22]

Our cave-dwelling ancestors slept in groups for

9

safety. This is still common practice in many tribal cultures when safety during sleep is needed (and possibly still in many houses around the world when those frightened by storms dash into another's bed for comfort). Many early civilisations adopted group sleep as a standard practice because it was practical and afforded people a time and place to socialise. To address the issue of keeping the species alive, a common feature of group sleep was that a man and a woman would come together in a bed for procreation only—more than likely one that afforded some privacy. This practice is identified in writings on Greek and Egyptian cultural practices.

The evolution of the bed itself started to influence whether individuals were able to enjoy the luxury of sleeping alone. The availability of a bed and bedroom for oneself was initially reliant on wealth and social status – and in places such as Britain, dependent upon how big your castle was. If you had no wealth, social status, or castle, you remained relegated to dorm-style sleeping facilities, or you might be lucky to have a pallet, trundle bed or bench in your lord's chamber. These conditions prevailed through the Middle Ages. The understanding from writings of those times is still the notion of group sleep as the norm with couples still coming together in a private space for procreation only.[23]

It wasn't until the late nineteenth century that regular bed-sharing for couples became more common. The Industrial Revolution brought families from the country into towns and this move presented them with houses that were much smaller than the spacious country-style homes they had left. Therefore, sharing a bed shifted from being something a couple might do to enjoy some conjugal rights, to being a non-negotiable, night-time reality. But this didn't mean that everyone was happy with the arrangement.

Despite the growing practice of bed-sharing, there were still social groups attached to the practice of sleeping separately. They did tend to be the wealthier members of society, who continued to uphold the notions of privacy and propriety found in a room of one's own.

The historical record reveals that sharing a bed is a recent cultural norm, with no science behind it. Posh people have never done it. It's a mark of wealth to sleep separately—it should be aspirational. It is said that "sensible Victorians are said to have wailed about the intolerable cruelty of having to share a bed".[24]

An episode of the popular Carnival Films (UK) drama *Downton Abbey,* set in Britain in the early 1900s, has a scene in which the lady of the manor is in bed, and her eldest daughter Mary (in her twenties and still living at home) is sitting talking to her. The Lord comes in wearing his bathrobe, prepared to come to bed. Mary asks her father, "Dad, could you at least pretend you sleep in separate beds like normal people?" He replies, "I keep a bed made up in my suite for the sake of propriety, and that's the most you should expect."

The ongoing evolution of the home has seen dwellings become more sophisticated and separated into designated areas for a specific use – e.g., eating, living, and sleeping. Cheaper housing materials and building methods have given families in developed Western societies, and middle to upper socio-economic groups access to more space. This has provided more opportunities for people to enjoy their own room if desired. However, cultural, social, and socioeconomic factors still impact on both the choice and the reality of whether you get a bed and a room to yourself each night.

Bundling

In the 16th and 17th Centuries there was a, what now seems a strange, custom of unmarried people sleeping the night together while fully clothed. The practice, called bundling, was said to have originated in rural parts of Wales or Scotland although it was most widespread in early America.

The few modern sources that that mention bundling describes it as a courtship ritual; lovers spent the night together in order to get to know each other. This, it is claimed was to ensure that they got on with each other because at the time divorce was not permitted and so a broken marriage had to be avoided. However, the idea that one night alone fully clothed on a bed was enough to ensure a stable marriage seems fanciful and indeed an early reference to bundling gives a different explanation. Grose, in his *Dictionary of the Vulgar Tongue* 1785, gives the following definition:

> *Bundling – 'A man and a woman lying on the same bed with their clothes on; an expedient practiced in America on a scarcity of beds, where, on such occasions, husbands and parents frequently permitted travelers to bundle with their wives and daughters'.*

While it is true that much later Webster in 1864 states that 'bundle' is "to sleep on the same bed without undressing; applied to the custom of a man and woman, especially lovers, thus sleeping", it can be seen that bundling was practised in two forms first, between strangers, as a simple domestic make-shift arrangement, often arising from the necessities of rural life and, secondly, as Stiles in 1871[25] puts it "between lovers, who shared the same couch, with the mutual understanding that innocent endearments should not be exceeded".

Essentially in past times, it was, for many reasons, dangerous to travel after dark and so strangers, or visiting lovers were permitted to share a bed, in a totally non-sexual manner, (one account describes the scandalous behaviour of a young woman who removed her outer garments before bundling). Thus, it was a simple expedience for a young man who had 'called' on his girlfriend to sleep in the family house rather than making them, perhaps, long journey home in the dark.

What is immutable and timeless across all cultures and civilisations is the reality that access to resources (property and money) always has and will determine the amount of space you have. In our homes, or wherever we look to lay our heads at night, there is more space and choice when we have more property and money. This is why an eight-bed dorm will always be the fate and domain of the budget traveller, and the multi-room hotel suite the destination of the wealthy.

Alongside the physical evolution of where we can sleep, social evolution has seen the bed shifting from a place of protection and procreation to a more private and intimate space for two people in a relationship.

The increases in moral and economic freedom seen since the middle of the twentieth century have certainly impacted on our night-time behaviours. Changing moral standards through the 1950s, '60s and '70s saw couples living together rather than marrying but enjoying all the benefits of a marriage, which include sleeping in a bed together.

And so, we arrive at today, where couples share a bed as the 'cool thing to do'. But history also tells us that this isn't the only configuration that is acceptable or possible, or more importantly, desirable. There appears to be no evidence to say that a couple in a bed each night is the deigned evolutionary track. We would suggest that all the evidence is to the contrary – it's what works for you and your cultural, social, and economic conditions.

Cultural contrast

Outside contemporary western society, many cultures ascribe a different meaning and importance to the 'who is where with whom and in what bed?' question. While there is a wealth of research into the science of sleep, there is a dearth of information when it comes to anthropological scrutiny over the behavioural aspect of sleeping. However, the following information provides some insight into the understanding that not all cultures view 'couple sleep' the same way.

African, Asian, and South American cultures approach sleep pragmatically, with some still preferring group sleepover private spaces. How the way each individual, family, social group or 'tribe' approaches sleeping is based more on local and inherited practices rather than broader social norms.

> As a couple, it's never really mattered where we sleep. Our kids have always slept with us or in our room – either on the bed or on the floor. In our family, we have Italian, Malay and Aboriginal heritage and the practice of the family sleeping in various places around the house has just always been the way we 'do life' in our house. This is common practice that has been in my family for generations. My daughter is now doing the same with her first child. Her husband is Islander, and they too have more a 'group' approach to who sleeps where.
>
> Dianne, 52, Educational Professional

Japan has a strong culture of couples sleeping in separate rooms. Jay Dwivedi, a commentator on Japanese culture, reports that as many as 70% of Japanese couples do not sleep together once they have a child. Before having a child, 25% of the couples do not sleep together. Despite being at an age when their libidos are running wild, *Shukan Bunshun*, a popular Japanese magazine, reports that as many as three out of four couples in their twenties prefer a separate bedroom.[26] Casey Baseel reported in 2013 that the lifestyle of husbands and wives in Japan is less integrated than in other countries, and this leads to an increase in a willingness or need to sleep separately. Baseel reported on a study from Hideki Kobayashi of Chiba University whose research found that 26% of married couples living in Tokyo-area condominiums sleep in separate rooms, four out of ten married couples over

60 don't share a bed, and that 53% of spouses whose children have moved out prefer to sleep solo.[27]

Marriages in which the couple do not live together are becoming increasingly common in modern Beijing, China. Guo Jianmei, director of the centre for women's studies at Beijing University, explains that "Walking marriages reflect sweeping changes in Chinese society".[28] This practice sees the husband in the couple 'walk' to his wife's family home if physical relations are sought, but with no day-to-day domestic life, nor sharing of property.

A similar arrangement exists in Saudi Arabia. It is called a *misyar* marriage and involves the husband and wife living separately but meeting regularly.

In comparison, a tribe in South Sudan (where polygamy operates) has a law that says husband and wife must sleep in the same bed. If couples don't sleep in the same bed, it is seen as a sign of marital unhappiness and can be interpreted as not wanting to have sex. In this male-dominated tribe, a woman refusing to sleep with her husband will result in elders and family members getting involved to try and solve 'the problem'. Exceptions do exist for such reasons as nursing babies, pregnancy, menstruation, or extreme sickness, but whatever the reason, the tribe always views the act of sleeping in separate beds as weakening the relationship.

If a wife does not sleep with her husband, there is something wrong with the marriage. It is the law that says man and wife should sleep together. If the woman does not sleep with the man, then the problem needs to be taken to the tribal elders and fixed. If my wife refuses to sleep in the same bed and

have sex with me, I think she is trying to punish me.
This can lead to divorce.
Abedi, 38, school teacher, married for 3 years

Religion and beds

While there do not appear to be many direct religious influences on the practice of sleeping in the same or separate beds, Klösch[29] notes that men and women sleeping together did not always suit the moral concepts of the church. In the Middle Ages, historian Einhard (circa AD830) warned that the bed was to provide shared accommodation for a man and a woman who were joined by love and should only be used for procreation.

Among Orthodox Jews, it is standard practice for married couples to have two beds because of Niddah (menstrual purity) laws. These laws forbid a married couple from touching each other for at least 12 days out of every menstrual cycle. To work around the laws, couples will have twin beds that they push together or pull apart as appropriate.[30]

The Koran instructs Muslim couples to sleep separately when one is committing nushuz. This is where one partner in a couple is, in essence, rebelling against the confines of the marriage. Until the issue is addressed, the Koran instructs husbands to 'avoid their wives in sleeping places...' (Koran 4:34).[31]

Some religions have dogmatic attitudes about a woman's place in marriage – namely that she is subservient to her

17

husband. This attitude could prevent, or at least limit, a woman's ability to be assertive enough to take steps to sleep separately or put enormous social pressure on her to accept 'her lot'. It would be reasonable to assume that religions that allow one partner a level of control over the other could influence sleeping arrangements if the dominant person of the couple decided that sharing the bed was something they wanted to do. However, there does not appear to be a religion that makes always sharing a bed compulsory.

> *A Christian mind set influences your view of marriage. Often people have engaged in Christian exchange of vows, so somewhere in their psyche and worldview is the belief that a woman belongs to a man. It's a possessive act to say 'this is where you will sleep' and my sense, when I hear women complaining about not sleeping, is that the women are contracted to that arrangement in such a way that makes it hard for them to challenge or change it. I think that their contract is emotional, sexual, economic, and religious, and I think it becomes too big to challenge it because it speaks of other things for both parties of a lack of voice, or a lack of opinion or 'who wears the pants'.*
> Neil, 46, HR Executive, married 19 years

Twin beds

> *...and so rode easily to Welling, where we supped well, and had two beds in the room and so lay single, and still remember it that of all the nights that ever*

*I slept in my life I never did pass a night with more
epicurism of sleep*
Samuel Pepys 23rd September 1661

Twin beds were a popular sleeping arrangement for
married couples between 1870 and 1970 and have
continued to be a ubiquitous piece of bedroom furniture
in many images of a decorous couple. But twin beds
have been written about for many years and espoused
as a healthy way to sleep.[32]

> *The twin-bed seems to have come to stay, and will
> no doubt in time succeed the double bed in all rooms
> occupied by two persons. As a matter of economy
> and space it is not practicable in every family that
> each member should have a separate room. But it
> is exceedingly desirable that each member should
> sleep in a separate bed. So high an authority as the
> Lancet, in a recent article, condemned the double
> bed as unwholesome. It said in effect that no two
> persons could sleep in this way regularly for a
> period of any length without one or the other feeling
> evil effects from it. The more lymphatic, robust
> person is sure to draw nervous force from the more
> delicate and more nervous person, end it is not
> uncommon for both to rise in the morning jaded and
> dull, whereas they would have risen refreshed and
> invigorated had they slept in separate beds. The twin
> beds offer a complete remedy for these evils, while
> they occupy but a trifle more space than the double
> bed. This twin arrangement consists of two beds
> which are intended to be placed side by side, and
> the design of which is usually incomplete unless they*

are so placed. A separate spring mattress and bed
clothing are provided for each bed, and the sleeper
enjoys the perfect restfulness of a separate bed.
Worthing Gazette – 12 October 1892

Propriety, modesty, and good hygiene came together in the ultimate solution of sharing a bedroom, while maintaining a sensible distance.

On this account, it is more wholesome to sleep single,
than double, for there is then less destruction of
oxygen; and the atmosphere is much purer and cooler.
Robert Macnish. The philosophy of sleep 1830

The majority of those who favoured twin beds said
they did so because of "incompatibility sleeping
habits"—differences in ideas on the amount of
bedclothes and restless and snoring husbands.
Daily Mirror 8 March 1939

Tiffs twin A wife with a bedroom problem writes to us
under the nom-de-plume "BALANCING BRIGHTON
IAN," Sussex: I have been married for a good many
years but am now just about fed-up with balancing
on six inches of the bed every night. When I suggest
twin beds, my husband just looks hurt and asks what
for; he says he's quite comfortable. What do other
wives do—go out and buy twin beds or just put up
with the discomfort? If any wife has succeeded in
swapping a double for twin beds lately and got away
with it without hurting her old man's feelings, we'll be
glad to hear how she did it!
Daily Mirror – 2 December 1959

The 1960s saw couples enticed by loosening social rules, developing freedom to express themselves, and birth control, which made sharing a bed a more popular choice. Confined now to the platonic travellers, twin beds have not made a resurgence – but come back in a decade or two, and who knows?

In good company

Even though sleeping apart can be a taboo subject, there are many famous people who are open about the practice and lead the way in debunking the myths thanks to the media's fascination of their sleeping behaviours.

The Queen of England and Prince Phillip were one of the most famous couples to sleep apart – they even had separate cabins on the Royal Yacht Britannia.[33] Seventy-three years of marriage would suggest that theirs was a successful union if longevity is anything to go by. Following their marriage, they moved into Clarence House in 1949 and had adjacent, connecting rooms. The Queen's cousin, Lady Pamela Mountbatten, explained, "You don't want to be bothered with snoring or someone flinging a leg around. When you are feeling cosy, you share your room sometimes. It is lovely to be able to choose." The Queen was not the only royal to confess to the practice. In October 2013 Princess Michael of Kent revealed that she slept in 'separate quarters' to her husband Prince Michael, so they were "fresher for each other", and Prince Michael of Kent claimed that spending time apart from his wife in general "made their marriage richer".[34] King Charles and

Camilla have continued the practice, reported (but not confirmed) to share three bedrooms – one each, and one to share, and Prince William and Princess Kate too, have separate sleeping arrangements to assist in being well rested to manage busy schedules. With all the space royal families have available in various residences... why wouldn't one?

And it's not just royalty that has taken themselves off to separate chambers.[35] Pop culture websites reported that during their marriage, Katie Holmes and Tom Cruise didn't share a bedroom due to Tom's snoring. Apparently, even Kevin Jonas, at the tender age of 23, sleeps separately from his wife, Danielle Deleasa, because of his snoring.[36] Scott Disick and Kourtney Kardashian were outed as separate sleepers in an episode of *Kourtney and Kim Take New York*. *E! Online* reported that the couple slept in separate beds. Disick explained, 'Just want to clear up the reason why we don't sleep in bed together. I'm not a good sleeper and with [son] Mason in bed I can't fall to sleep!"

And during their marriage, Kim and Kanye (Ye) spent sleeping time apart so Kanye would have enough sleep to keep him functioning creatively. Allegedly, Kim's second pregnancy was particularly difficult and saw them head to separate rooms.

Our most divisive American President Donald Trump is a famous separate sleeper also. I'm sure not many people would blame Melania for wanting time away from his reported incessant TV watching and late-night snacking. Maybe Trump took his cues from the Netflix show *House of Cards*. Kevin Spacey and Robyn Wright as President and First Lady parted company each night in the 'White House' heading across the corridor to separate bedrooms.

Australian producer Baz Luhrmann and wife Catherine Martin cite intense contact by working together as the reason they head to separate rooms.[37] "We worked out a long time ago that we both need space. We are surrounded by our teams of staff all day every day, whether travelling, at work and at our homes. I was finding I was saying things in passing that weren't properly thought through, things would become fraught. We both needed time to ourselves." To keep the spark in their relationship, Luhrmann says they do 'Saturday night hotel dates', spending the next day relaxing, not heading home until the afternoon.

Then there are the couples who take sleeping apart to the next level by sleeping in separate houses. Mia Farrow and Woody Allen maintained separate apartments across New York's Central Park for a number of years.[38] People could argue that this distance may have had some impact on the events that unravelled their marriage— we'll never know. In 2019 Gwyneth Paltrow and Brad Falchuk[39] explained that they spend half of each week in separate houses – citing get a good night's sleep as one of the motivations for choosing this arrangement. Sandra Bullock and partner Bryan Randall are reported[40] to head to separate beds as 'getting a full night's sleep is almost a religion for Sandra'. Separate sleeping arrangements have been in place for every relationship of Bullock's due to 'strict routines in her life', which include prioritising sleep.

Victoria and David Beckham have also taken the path of separate living quarters with report that their country home has distinct 'his and her' wings. According to reports, each wing has its own kitchen, bedrooms, and courtyard.

'It works out well for David, Victoria, and the kids. If they are all driving each other mad, they can retreat into these wings like they are living in separate houses.'

Another couple that decided separate 'wings' in a house was 'the go' is Sarah Jessica Parker and Matthew Broderick. For them, this involved tearing down a wall of adjoining town houses in New York, with each of them taking one side and their children having access to both. Apparently, this setup was partly designed as a compromise of Parker's neat lifestyle and Broderick's messy one. But despite the separated accommodations, the source was clear that the couple continues to spend quality time together and even have the occasional 'sleepover'.

Social Media

Separate sleeping or a 'sleep divorce' is trending topic on both Reddit and TikTok. There are various conversations within relationship and r/AskReddit Subreddits about separate sleeping. The conversations are focussed on who sleeps separately and if it's normal. There are also many people sharing their 'Sleep Divorce' stories or talking about the pros and cons of 'sleep divorces' in the ubiquitous short videos of TikTok. We think this is great news as the younger demographic of the platform may approach the separate sleeping conversation with less hesitancy if they have seen relatable 'bites' of information about it.

So why do we sleep together?

In a paper[41] considering if sleep was an activity worthy of sociological consideration, Brian Taylor suggests that we stop talking about 'being asleep' and start talking about 'doing sleeping'. His reason for this suggestion is that he proposes a 'discourse of dormancy' be created that truly brings sleep into the sociological domain. It seems that Taylor underestimates the vast number of conversations already taking place between couples and families across the world about how they 'do sleeping'.

The problem is though that these conversations are not in the public domain – they are in the shared bedrooms of the world. Scientific research has focused mostly on how individuals sleep every night, while in bedrooms around the world, social experiments in sleeping together are being conducted every night. The discourse of 'will you stop that; I can't get to sleep' has been part of our language for a long time and isn't about to stop any time soon.

While we have provided an overview of the social history of sleep, it is important to understand that the current western culture expectation of sleeping with your partner every night is a relatively new phenomenon, as is the idea that sleeping together is somehow an indicator of the strength, or otherwise, of the relationship. However, an historical and anthropological perspective provides a different view on the real reason some of us sleep together and why it is not necessarily 'natural' or 'normal' to do so.

Humans are the only animals that chose to sleep together for 'intimacy'. Other animals sleep together for warmth and/or security or because of physical proximity. Animals choose their 'sleep sites', e.g., nest in the tree, in an underground burrow or a cave, because of their need for warmth or security. Our early ancestors would have had the same considerations in mind when choosing where they slept. Because they were hunter-gatherers, therefore by nature nomadic, they had to be able to transport their entire life with them, and that almost certainly did not involve lugging a bed around with them. They would sleep, close but safely, near to what every activity they were carrying out.

However, while they may have pretty much slept anywhere since time immemorial man has made preparation for sleep to make our 'sleep site' as comfortable as possible; for instance, laying an animal pelt on the ground or using plant matter as some sort of mattress (often using certain plants specifically to produce a nice smell or to keep bugs at bay). This peripatetic lifestyle and need for comfort are mirrored in the behaviour of our closest cousins the great apes who do not sleep in the same place twice. Each night they make a new nest, and it has been observed that if the nest is not comfortable, they will either modify the nest or make an entirely new one. Adults also do not share a bed.

Originally, we would have all slept together on the ground mainly because we had nowhere else from which to choose, but we would have also chosen warmth and security. Even in early Tudor times, the poor slept on the floor; men, women, children, animals, and even passing travellers all bedded down together near, but not too near the fire. Most 'houses' until the 15th century were simple constructions with a fire in the middle of the main room, with the smoke from the fire escaping through holes, obviously small, in the roof. This design was necessary because the building materials used at this time were flammable. However, one drawback of these 'hall' houses was that that the upper parts of the house would have been very smoky and it is for this reason that it was not possible to have a habitable second floor to the house.

Therefore, it was only when we started using non-flammable building materials to build our houses, which specifically allowed us to construct chimneys to vent the smoke, that people were able to create another floor in their homes giving them the extra space to construct the 'bedroom'. The additional space in the bedroom gave us the ability to erect permanent, rope framed, beds upon which we could then put our mattresses. This also provided additional protection from crawling biting things. Often, if space allowed, two bedrooms would be constructed, one for the numerous children and one for the parents and any newborn child.

This sleeping arrangement caused merely by lack of space, has led to our idea that sleep, sex, and the bedroom are somehow linked. In other animals there is no connection between sleep and sex, they are entirely separate activities carried out at different times and different locations, and indeed humans are the only animals who explicitly choose to have sex where they sleep. The reason they became linked in the human mind is that at the same time as we started building 'bedrooms' we were also developing our sense of shame/embarrassment. Therefore, because sleep and sex were behind the closed bedroom door, as it was the one place the adults could get some privacy, the bedroom became inextricably linked with sleep and sex.

But our ideas of sleep and sex seem rather confused in that we use the phrase 'sleeping together' to mean both activities (I always thought that it was impolite to fall asleep during sex!). This link between sleep and sex became most closely linked in the Victorian times when the double bed symbolised the "extraordinary Victorian commitment to reproduction" leading to the assertion that "the output of the factory was less important, in the long run than that of the double bed" Esme Wingfield-Stratford 'The Victorian Tragedy'. However, in the late nineteenth and early 20th century, there was a move away from double beds to identical twin beds or two separate beds, one large for intimacy and another smaller bed either in the same room or in an adjacent room when one partner desired solitude.

Thus, sleeping together is essentially a modern phenomenon brought about by our humble dwellings and is not in any way the natural order of things. Indeed, through history, it has only ever been the poor who have slept together because of space limitations. The rich, on the other hand, had the space to be able to adopt any sleeping arrangements that worked for them. They had beds of ever-increasing elaboration, comfort, and expense but again until comparatively recently however big their castle they did not specifically have a bedroom instead their bed travelled around with them and was put up in a suitable room wherever they happened to be staying that night.

Of course, this is very much from the European perspective; many cultures have not found it necessary to adopt the idea of sleeping together. However, it is perfectly natural for the mother to share a bed with their child, to provide warmth, food, security, and love. For most of the world's population, this is a perfectly normal state of affairs with even quite old children still sharing the mothers, or more rarely parents, bed. This is perhaps not the place to discuss the 'scientific' view of this behaviour, but one should note that humans are the only animal where, some, parents sleep together to the exclusion of the child.

A Sleep Divorce

The last two years have seen the rise of the term 'Sleep Divorce'[42] – mentioned early as a trending topic on Tiktok. Even though we have titled the book 'A Sleep Divorce' we both find the term somewhat misleading for the practice of sleeping separately – and we are not alone in our dislike of the term. The simple definition of 'divorce' is inexorably linked the end of a marriage, or in more neutral terms 'to separate or dissociate something from something else, typically with an undesirable effect' – and for so many couples, separate sleeping brings about an opposite outcome – often bringing them closer together.

Another common connotation of the term 'divorce' is that it's an unhappy, final ending of a relationship. Again – a couple choosing to sleep separately are not ending their marriage in an unhappy way. In fact, the choice might even elicit the opposite in both regards.

We suggest that couples who are choosing to sleep

separately because they are ending their marriage might be advised to read a different book as providing advice in that area is outside the realm of our expertise.

We believe that the term 'sleep divorce' has gained traction as it's headline-grabbing and provocative. However, we also understand the need to find a 'usable' phrase to describe a new practice or concept, so are both beginning to reluctantly accept that the term is making its way into common parlance, and maybe we need to get on board.

We do both remain quizzical as to what's wrong with simply stating 'we're sleeping separately'? No divorce needed – just a good night's sleep; thank you very much.

Pause for thought...

- Are you aware that a couple sleeping by themselves in a shared bed in a bedroom was a relatively new western-culture phenomenon?
- Are you aware of what the sleeping arrangements of your parents or grandparents, or older friends and relatives, are or were? If so, what are they?
- Are you aware of any sleeping arrangements by friends or relatives that challenge the norm of a couple sleeping in the same bed together? If so, what are they?
- Do you have any preconceived ideas about who should sleep with whom in specific social arrangements? Do you ever talk about these to others, or judge other people because of their choices?

- Do you know anyone whose sleeping arrangements are dictated by cultural or religious expectations?
- Do you or your partner have cultural or religious influences that impact how you think about or manage your sleeping arrangements? If so, what are they?
- Do you ever talk to other people about any sleep-related issues? Is it common to do so in your social groups?

TWO

The Science of Sleep

'If you didn't know what sleep was, and you had only seen it in a science fiction movie, you would think it was weird and tell all your friends about the movie you'd seen.

George Carlin[43]

If you have been sharing a bed for ten weeks, ten months or ten years and wonder why you feel or look ten years older than you are, then lack of sleep could be the reason. Just as biomechanics is essential for those who exercise, and food science needs to be understood for those who diet, the science behind sleep is a crucial factor to consider in the domain of bed-sharing.

The physiology of sleep differs from person to person. Factors that impact on how our body manages sleep are hardwired into each individual's DNA and are not necessarily open for negotiation. As couples we all accept that we are not always going to like the same food, exercise at the same time (if at all), have the same religious beliefs or the same tastes in television shows. So why do we think that our sleep needs are going to be similar? Or do we even think about sleep when we set out to find a partner?

Who includes sleeping behaviours in the list of 'must-haves' when considering a dream partner? Was it ever on your list? Did you ever think, 'He needs to be at least six-feet tall, handsome, dark hair, love the outdoors and need at least seven hours of sleep each night, going to bed somewhere between 9 and 10 pm.' Similarly, it is doubtful if "so tell me about your circadian rhythms and melatonin production cycle" has been a popular conversation starter at speed dating events in bars and nightclubs.

A problem with shared sleeping in blossoming relationships is that in the early days, it is often an activity of low importance. The chemicals of attraction that see us pursuing another will send couples into a blissful daze, with the practicalities of daily life ignored in favour of the more exciting activities of a new relationship. Remember, when you were young, you could sleep in a single bed snuggled up to your beloved. However, every relationship eventually moves into the everyday. And it is in the routine and potential monotony of life that every relationship begins to face its challenges. Once a couple starts heading to bed most nights just to sleep – rather than tear each other's clothes off with unbridled passion – is when the harsh necessities of this nightly human activity reveal their true impact.

While this book focuses on helping couples maintain

their relationships despite different sleep needs, the bitter reality is that without enough sleep, we can all begin to fall apart as a person. We all need enough rest every day to give us the mental, emotional, and physical strength to manage our lives. And if you are in a situation when you aren't having this each night – whatever the reason – then you might find yourself 'falling apart' both on a personal level and a relationship level.

Jennifer's lack of sleep, and the effect it had on her physically, emotionally, and mentally, led her to thinking about the activity of sleep – a bit obsessively at times, she admits. When she was not getting enough sleep, she turned to research to help her understand why she felt so physically awful and mentally inept. After reading about sleep deprivation, she remembers feeling a strong sense of relief that the symptoms she was experiencing, such as irritability, low energy, and lack of concentration, were neither uncommon nor inconsequential.

So why all this fuss about sleep?

Without any question or doubt, human beings need sleep. Why we need sleep is a question that has challenged scientists for centuries. The earliest documented sleep theory is attributed to the Greek philosopher and physician Alcmaeon in 500–450 BC who wrote about blood flow in the sleeping body.[44]

The scientific community admits that no definitive explanation exists about why we need to sleep despite the time spent exploring the question. What is understood and known though, is that sleep is an anabolic, or building process, that has a range of positive effects on the human body.

Positive effects of sleep

Sleep has numerous positive effects on the body[45], including:

- conserving and restoring the body's energy supplies that have been depleted through the day's activities
- providing a time for the body to do most of its repair work; muscle tissue is rebuilt and restored
- allowing for the secretion of growth hormone, which is vital for growth in children, and also crucial throughout adulthood to rebuild tissues
- restoring mental energy; we spend all day thinking and creating and using our energy stores, and sleep replenishes these stores
- providing downtime for changes in the structure and organisation of the brain, a phenomenon known as brain plasticity
- inducing the production of collagen and enhancing the skin's capacity to hold water, which are two key ingredients to keeping your skin as close as possible to your chronological age
- reinforcing memory and learning by allowing the brain to replay the events of the day
- improving immune responses.

The benefits of sleep are a good reason alone to get your

eight hours every night. Although why we sleep is not definitively understood, there is no dispute among sleep researchers about what happens when we don't get enough sleep.

A lack of sleep has serious effects on our ability to function.[46] Countless studies have shown that humans struggle to function if sleep deprived. The 3rd edition of the International Classification of Sleep Disorders distinguished nearly one hundred different sleep disorders – so there's no shortage of information on what can go wrong. There are sleep laboratories in most countries that research what we should and shouldn't be doing when it comes to sleep and an increasing stream of findings from sleep research about the effects of too much, not enough, or unusual sleeping patterns in humans.

Of particular interest is a recurrent finding in sleep research that when it comes to sleeping – like so many other parts of our life – men and women are different. While we are wary that this book might portray men as the villains of sleep disturbance, research findings aren't in their favour (sorry guys!). Klösch reports that studies have found only minor biological differences between men and women when it comes to how we sleep.[47] However, a 2007 study titled 'Sex differences in the reactions to sleeping in pairs versus sleeping alone in humans' reported more discernible differences in the impact men have on women when they share a bed.[48]

The study investigated what the actual and perceived effects of sleeping with a partner were for both men and women. John Dittami, the lead author of the study, found, 'the bottom line is that our results indicate that women are more disturbed by the male presence in bed than the men by a woman's presence. When it came to the perceived effects, he concluded that 'women enjoy male presence psychologically even though it costs them minutes or even hours of sleep'. There are behaviours where men are represented more prominently than women in the sport of 'waking up my partner'. These behaviours will be discussed in chapter three.

Discussions with couples over the last five years would support the findings anecdotally, but certainly not exclusively, as you will see throughout the book. We are all aware that there are many physiological differences between genders. This is just another of those areas of difference that when approached sensibly, can be noted and managed.

Issues such as sleep patterns, environmental needs and temperature issues consistently highlight an arena for the 'battle of the sexes' to continue its tournament of differences. As an example, one commonly reported gender difference is found in the contest of the light versus the heavy sleeper. Klösch[49] explains that because of biological, cultural, and social conditions, women are disposed to an increased need to control their environment, which contributes to issues with falling asleep and staying asleep as they are more sensitive to any stimuli that might wake them. In contrast, men tend to avoid or ignore stimuli and fall asleep as soon as their heads hit the pillow.

A 2012 study by the Appleton Institute at the Central Queensland University, called the 'Sealy Sleep Census Report',[50] surveyed over 13,000 people and found that males fall asleep on average eleven minutes faster than females, and seem to be mostly untroubled after that.

*Storms, pets, phones, neighbours ... nothing wakes
my husband up. I would love to have his skill of
putting my head on the pillow and being asleep in
a nanosecond like he does. Honestly, I think I could
take another man into bed, and he wouldn't notice.*
Lulu, 42, legal professional, married 6 years

*I've given up on expecting him to wake up when
the kids need something during the night. I quite
amaze myself how I can hear the slightest noise from
the other end of the house. Maybe it's a superhero
power I've developed. Don't think I will become
famous for it, though.*
Maria, 38, database analyst, married 8 years

*I don't think I will revert back to where we were in
the beginning with our sleeping, even when the
children have grown up. I do expect that my sleeping
will permanently be changed from having children
and always listening out for them. I expect I will be
sleeping by myself a few nights a week forever now.*
Maree, 30, health professional, married 3 years

To further support that gender differences are indeed an
issue for many couples and backing up the 2007 study
by Dittami on sex differences in sleep, a 2010 survey by
The National Sleep Foundation[51] found that more than
half the women they surveyed, aged 18 to 64, said they
slept well only a few nights a week because of sharing a
bed. Of these, 43% believed their lack of sleep interfered
with their ability to deal with the next day's activities.

After two years of not sleeping properly due to my

partner's snoring and movement in bed, I couldn't function anymore. Every day I was cranky with everyone and reached the point where I felt like I was falling apart. I started to put on weight, would go to work with an aching body, and couldn't cope with the normal pressures of life. My judgement was impaired to the point that I was so hypersensitive; I thought I was never going to sleep again.

Louise, 48, teacher, defacto for 7 years

Grumpy, irritable, indecisive, throwing tantrums ... behaviour of a two-year-old, right? No, this is, in fact, me on many given days: a 28-year-old woman that should know how to act better. But it is literally beyond my control. This is how I act when I don't get enough sleep. I have a foggy mind; I cannot concentrate, am incredibly irritable, sometimes even shaky ... it's almost like having an awful hangover every day. I remember clearly one day being so tired and getting ready for work. Suddenly I wondered what the burning sensation under my arms was only to realise that instead of deodorant I had in fact sprayed hairspray all over myself!

Emily, 30, international flight attendant, married 4 years

My husband recently talked to me about not feeling very close anymore. I was surprised by his question, but then he told me that I had been telling him to f*** off for the past week when he tried to tuck me in and cuddle me after I went to my bed. I had no idea I was doing it – I'm just so tired. I felt so bad because the cuddles when I go to my bed are really important to us.

Charlotte, 24, teacher, married 1 year

Why men fall asleep after sex, after a big meal and in front of the TV

The feeling of being safe and secure is the reason why men fall asleep after sex and a large meal. From an evolutionary point of view, a man's role is primarily to hunt and to protect. Once he has provided food and ensured the safety of the group, there is little else useful for him to do – therefore he sleeps.

Now, for most animals, sleep and sex are not linked in any way because when you have sex, you are vulnerable, your back is turned, and your mind is on other things, so animals have sex very quickly. Therefore, if a man feels safe and secure enough to have nice, pleasurable sex then he is also safe and secure enough to go to sleep and as he has had a hard day hunting and protecting and because sleep is so important, he will go to sleep.

The same is true with regards eating when you have your head stuck in a wildebeest's carcass you are vulnerable. Hence, you either take your food somewhere safe or you eat quickly, thus if you are safe and secure enough to have a nice pleasurable meal you are safe and secure enough to sleep. And the same rings true with the TV – if you are relaxed enough to be able to watch the game in peace again it gives the signal you are safe and secure, so you can fall asleep.

For both genders, just one night without sleep makes concentration more difficult and shortens our attention span considerably. With continued lack of sleep, the part of the brain that controls language, memory, planning and sense of time is severely affected, practically shutting down. In fact, an Australian study in 1997[52] discovered that only seventeen hours of sustained wakefulness leads to a decrease in performance equivalent to a blood alcohol level of 0.05% – two glasses of wine and the legal driving limit in many countries.

Research also shows that sleep-deprived individuals often have difficulty in responding to rapidly changing situations and in making rational judgements. In real-life situations, the consequences are grave, and lack of sleep is said to have been a contributing factor to such infamous disasters as the Exxon Valdez oil spill, the Chernobyl and Three Mile Island nuclear reactor meltdowns, and the Challenger shuttle explosion.[53]

The accidents stemming from lack of sleep are not limited to large-scale catastrophes. Bob Ellis, an Australian political commentator, has noted many political career-threatening (and ending) decisions and actions by Australian politicians that he claims were due to sleep deprivation caused by plane flights. He includes Australian Prime Minister Julia Gillard's 2010 gaff in Geneva when she declared that foreign policy 'was not her passion', and the Leader of the Opposition Tony Abbott declaring at the same time in Afghanistan that 'shit happens' when asked about his thoughts on soldiers dying in the course of their duties.[54] Neither statement set them in a winning political position but instead left a public relations disaster for their media staff to clean up.

Although most of us do not have jobs as important as head of state, there are times when all of us can recall putting in less than stellar performances at work or even in our relationships when in a sleep-deprived state.

My wife was due to give birth and was not sleeping well.

Her tossing and turning kept us both awake for about two weeks straight. At the time, I was in charge of entering data into a database used to calculate university entrance scores of the senior students at the school where I worked. It was only the request of the Head of English for a copy of the grade's scores entered for the subject that saved the students from a catastrophe. When entering the data, I had skipped a name at the top of the list and entered all remaining scores incorrectly. In my tired state, I hadn't even picked up that I was 'out of sync' when I got to the end of the list. My mistake would have significantly impacted many students' lives, and I hadn't even realised.

Warren, 52, deputy principal

Consequences of sleep deprivation

Sleep deprivation can lead to[55]:

- fatigue, lethargy, and lack of motivation
- moodiness and irritability
- reduced creativity and problem-solving skills
- inability to cope with stress
- high blood pressure
- weakened immune system
- reduced ability to concentrate
- weight gain
- cosmetic signs of premature ageing
- increased risk of obesity
- impaired motor skills and increased risk of accidents
- difficulty making decisions

- increased risk of diabetes
- increased risk of heart disease
- memory loss
- possible episodes of sleep paralysis that are usually accompanied by hallucinations
- increased likelihood of mentally 'stalling' or fixating on one thought
- increased chance of becoming depressed.

On the issue of weight alone, a large US survey[56] in 1984 revealed that people who averaged six hours of sleep per night were 27% more likely to be overweight than those who got seven to nine hours. And those who averaged only five hours of sleep per night were 73% more likely to be overweight due to an imbalance in hormones that promote hunger – in particular, for simple sugars and carbohydrates – and a slowing down in the body's metabolic rate.

Since my husband and I moved into separate rooms, I am sleeping so much better. Because of the unbroken and better quality sleep, I'm getting up three mornings a week at 5.30am and exercising for an hour. Before we moved into separate rooms, I felt drained in the mornings; now I feel so rested and have energy to exercise. I'm actually losing weight.
Anne, 44, senior manager, married 20 years

I'm a very light sleeper, and my girlfriend is a restless sleeper who gets up, on average, about 3 hours earlier than I do. After 6 months of sleep-deprivation hell, I did gained weight – not too much, but enough to get me worried. We now sleep in separate rooms.
meepster00001, www.slate.com

A 2010 study[57] by the Woolcock Institute of Medical Research in Australia found that during deep sleep, metabolically active hormones, such as growth hormones, are secreted. People who don't fall into deep sleep, for example, people with sleep apnoea, don't get this growth hormone secreted, and this can increase the risk of obesity and diabetes.

How much sleep do you need?

As well as knowing why we need sleep and what happens when we don't, there is also the question of how much sleep each person needs. Even though there is a general acceptance that we need eight hours sleep a night (drummed into most of us since we were young), there appears to be no magic number. Just like many other unique characteristics we inherit at birth, the amount of sleep we need to function at our best varies among those who are of similar age, gender, ethnic or cultural group. Interestingly, some cultures view sleep as a waste of time and consider those people who function with minimal sleep as diligent and strong-willed.

Klösch[58] speaks of historical writings in China, Japan, and Europe, extolling the virtues of the political and clerical elite who required only a few hours of sleep. The similarity of God, who 'neither slumbers nor sleeps' (Psalm 121:3–4), to the person who could rule and lead with minimal rest each night, made eight hours each night the domain of wimps.

While some people can function on minimal amounts of sleep each night, most of us tend to need a little more. If you are a person who needs a good eight hours sleep every night and is wondering why you aren't one of these superheroes who can survive on a few paltry hours of sleep each day, stop giving yourself a hard time (especially given the fact that Adolf Hitler and Ghengis Kahn were also short sleepers). Researchers at the University of California, San Francisco,[59] discovered that some people have a gene that enables them to function on only a few hours of sleep a night. But the gene is very rare, appearing in less than 3% of the population; for the other 97% of us, it's six hours plus each night. So put the Lycra suit away and keep your underpants on the inside.

And if you are still feeling like an underperformer because you need more than four hours a night, take heart in knowing that Albert Einstein is reported to have required ten hours sleep each night to be well-rested and ready to solve those tricky scientific problems. (Neil would like to point out here that he also needs about 9.5-10 hours' sleep a night)

The common consensus from sleep researchers[60] is that most healthy adults need between seven to nine hours of sleep each day, although anywhere between three to eleven hours can be considered healthy depending on individual needs.

So how much sleep do I need?

The idea that we all need about eight hours of sleep a night is a myth. Individual sleep need is like height – we are all different, and some people need much more than eight hours while others need less. Anywhere between three and eleven hours is considered normal. Your sleep need is, to a large extent, genetically determined and getting less than your personal sleep need is a problem. Even having just one hour less sleep a night than you require can have measurable effects on your physical and mental health.

Good sleep means that we feel and function better during the day because, during sleep, our bodies and brain are given the opportunity to recover from the stress and strains of the day. During sleep, the brain processes the day's experiences deals with the emotional aspects of the day and memories are stored or eliminated.

Your sleep need is essentially the amount of sleep that allows you to feel awake, refreshed, and healthy during the following day. Very simply if you feel sleepy during the day, then you are probably not, for whatever reason, getting the sleep you need during the night. However, sleepy is not the same as tired/exhausted/ fatigued (although they may be a result of being sleepy), the question to ask yourself is if you climb three flights of stairs, do you need a sit-down or a sleep. If you need a sit-down, you are tired, fatigued, etc. but if you need a sleep, then you are sleepy.

Hopefully, this discussion is leading you to begin to understand that sleep is not quite as simple or straightforward as we may think. The complex nature of sleep has been researched extensively to help us understand more about what sleep is and how we (as humans) DO sleep. Sleep is not an activity that is the same for everyone. The complex relationship of systems in our bodies means that sleep is not the same experience for everyone. The following information aims to explain why how we 'do sleep' is so individual.

What is Sleep?

Sleep is regulated by two body systems, sleep/wake homeostasis and our circadian rhythm (a.k.a. 'body clock'). Sleep/wake homeostasis tells us how long we've been awake and at the end of the day tells us that it is time to get some to sleep. Our circadian rhythm regulates sleepiness and wakefulness over a 24-hour period. The circadian rhythm rises and falls across the day with our strongest sleep drive generally occurring between 2:00-4:00 am. There is also another dip in the afternoon between 1:00-3:00 pm, the so-called 'post-lunch dip', which because being a function of our circadian rhythm, does not need food for it to occur. Our circadian rhythm dictates whether we are a 'morning person' or 'evening person' and thus the exact timing of our peaks and troughs of alertness and sleepiness across the day. Essentially our body knows 'it's time for bed' when it goes dark as we produce a hormone called melatonin, which sets off a train of events that leads us to sleep.

Melatonin levels drop overnight, and in the morning our body clock starts a series of changes—increase in body temperature, production of the hormone cortisol— that signals it is time to get up. The body starts preparing to wake up about one hour before you, in fact, awake, hence if the body knows when you are going to wake, because you have set the alarm or because, as recommended, you have a regular wake up time, it can actually prepare to wake up at that time, hence your 'uncanny' ability to wake up before your alarm goes off. However, if it does not know when you are going to wake, it cannot prepare, and thus you are liable to feel groggy when you wake.

47

This can be a significant issue when sharing a bed each night with someone who has a different body clock to you, so they wake you each morning before you are physiologically ready to awaken.

The primary external signal that day has arrived is light. Just a few minutes of daylight is enough to tell the body that it is daytime. Even through closed eyes, light signals that it is time to wake up, hence we often in summer, we wake early. Because of our dependency on light/dark to entrain our body clock, our sleep need varies with the seasons. In summer we have a natural tendency to sleep less and in winter when it is dark and cold, we tend to sleep more.

Humans, in common with most animals, have evolved to sleep at night and be awake during the day. One of the main reasons for us to sleep at night is that our nocturnal vision is comparatively inferior; thus, we are unable to do anything at night usefully. Also, this means that we are vulnerable to predation, and hence it was best from a survival point of view to find somewhere safe at night and sleep. Our nocturnal vulnerability to being eaten by big hairy things with large teeth and good nocturnal vision also means that we can only sleep when we feel safe and secure.

Are you a lark or an owl?

Benjamin Franklin told us *"Early to bed and early to rise, makes a man healthy, wealthy, and wise"*.[61] But was he correct in his statement?

Do you find yourself wanting to go to sleep relatively

early and having no problem getting up early and feeling 'bright-eyed and bushy-tailed' and eager to start the day? If you answered 'yes', you're probably a lark. If you answered 'no' then you're probably an owl. Owls want to go to bed late and struggle to get up and out of bed first thing in the morning.

Morning-ness (a.k.a. 'lark') and evening-ness (a.k.a. 'owl') are in no small part genetically determined and although the timing of our sleep can be dictated by such external factors as our jobs, the primary external influence on the circadian rhythm—and therefore you're retiring and raising time—is light and dark.

For example, if you're an owl going to bed too early, because you are going against your circadian rhythm, you are going to find it harder to fall asleep. Because our circadian rhythm is, to a large degree genetically determined you cannot 'train' yourself to be a lark or an owl, although you can reduce the effects. For instance, owls would benefit from getting exposure to daylight as soon as possible after they wake up. Larks may find that getting out in the daylight late afternoon/early evening helps them to stay awake longer.

What's involved in Sleeping?

Sleep is divided into two distinct states—Rapid Eye Movement (REM) and non-REM sleep with non-REM sleep, traditionally being further divided into four stages, each of increasing depth. During the night, you pass through the four sleep stages: N1, N2, N3 and REM sleep in what is known as 'sleep cycles'. These stages progress cyclically from N1 through to REM then begin again with stage N1, with each sleep cycle lasting an average of 90 to 110 minutes. The first couple of sleep cycles of the night have long periods of deep N3 sleep with relatively short REM periods and later in the night; the REM periods lengthen and slow-wave sleep (SWS) is mostly absent. Thus the first third of the night is predominantly deep sleep while the latter part of the night is spent in stages N1 and N2 of non-REM sleep and in REM sleep.

Stage N1 (3-7% of sleep) is the lightest stage of sleep and is the transition between wake and sleep. It is the sleep that you have at the start of the night when you feel you are drifting in and out of sleep. When you are in stage N1 sleep, you can be wakened easily and indeed if you are awakened you will probably claim not to have been asleep. In stage N1, your eyes move slowly back and forth, and muscle activity reduces. At the transition from wake to sleep, many people experience sudden muscle contractions or jerks; a sensation of falling or a 'presence', benign or otherwise, in the room. It is also in stage N1 sleep that you are dipping in and out of when you wake in the middle of the night and feel you have been awake for hours.

In Stage N2 (45-50% of sleep) the slow-rolling eye movements seen in stage 1 sleep stop and your brain waves become slower with only an occasional burst of rapid brain waves. Although stage N2 sleep is the largest single portion of sleep, it is the stage about which we know least. In stage N3 sleep becomes deeper, slow brain waves (called delta waves) start to appear. Stages N3 (20-25% of sleep) is often referred to as 'deep' sleep or slow-wave sleep (SWS).

As is suggested by its name, when someone is in SWS, it can be very difficult to wake them. SWS is believed to be most closely linked with the restorative process of sleep and is the part of sleep that makes you feel you have had a good sleep. It also plays an important role in making you feel well-rested and energetic during the day. Research has shown that SWS is vital for memory and learning, and it is for this reason that children have proportionally more SWS than adults. This is also because SWS is the only time that you physically grow. It is during SWS that some people, particularly children, experience behaviours (known as parasomnias) such as bedwetting, sleep talking, sleepwalking or night terrors. Short and long sleepers essentially have the same amount of SWS thus a minimum amount of deep sleep is needed no matter how long is the total sleep time. Given the importance of SWS after partial or total sleep deprivation, the brain attempts to make up all the missed SWS.

In Rapid Eye Movement (REM) Sleep, (20-25% of sleep), the eyes jerk rapidly back and forth under closed eyelids, hence its name. It is during REM sleep that most 'story-like' dreams occur. Everyone dreams every night, and we have three to five periods of REM sleep each night; however, we can only remember a dream if we are woken during, or within a couple of minutes after it has finished. Therefore, if you do not wake during a dream, you will not remember it. REM sleep in involved in processing emotional memories and ensuring our psychological health. When we are dreaming the dream is, for all intents and purposes, real to both our mind and body and indeed our brain waves during this REM can increase to levels experienced when a person is awake. Also, during a dream, our breathing becomes more rapid, irregular, and shallow, heart rate increases, and blood pressure rises; essentially, we are 'living the dream'. However, so that we do not act out our dreams we are prevented from doing so by the fact that when we are in REM, we lose muscle tone and thus we are effectively paralysed for the duration of the dream. During REM, males may develop erections; however, this has nothing to do with the content of the dream and everything to do with simple fluid dynamics.

Opposite is a representation of a pretty good night's sleep showing the distribution of the various sleep stages across the night. Generally, in adults, most SWS occurs in the first third of the night with REM sleep happening approximately every 90 minutes throughout the night. Your first REM period may only be a matter of minutes long, but subsequent periods can be more than 30 minutes long. However good sleep is both quantity and quality, i.e., it is essential to get the right proportion and distribution of the various sleep stages during the night, that your sleep is as far as possible unbroken and that you get the sleep that is of the correct duration for you.

Sleep as We Age

It is untrue that people need less sleep as they grow older. What happens is that our sleep becomes less refreshing as we get older. This is because we get less of the deep, more restorative, stages of sleep and thus sleep is more

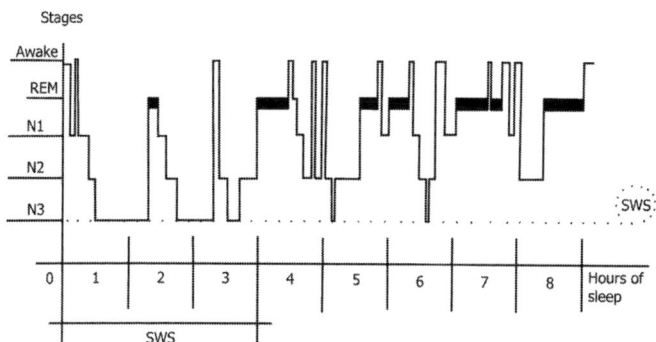

Stages

Awake | REM | N1 | N2 | N3

0 1 2 3 4 5 6 7 8 Hours of sleep

SWS

SWS

easily disturbed, even in healthy older people. When we are young, we fall asleep quickly and sleep soundly, but as we grow older people this loss of SWS makes sleep makes getting to sleep more difficult, we may awaken more often and then take longer to fall back to sleep.

Our sleep need becomes fixed in early adulthood and does not substantially change, even as we get older. So, while our sleep patterns may change over time, the need for sleep remains the same.

As we progress into middle age, although the duration of sleep we need to get remains pretty much the same as when we were 20, we start to lose our SWS per night progressively, and consequently, our sleep becomes less refreshing. This loss of deep sleep is most profound in men and generally starts around their mid-30s-40s while women start losing theirs in their 50s. This lack of refreshment from sleep causes many older people to feel that they are suffering from sleeping problems, whereas much of what they feel could be accounted for by the natural changes in their sleep.

This loss of deep sleep also means that we are more easily woken during the night, and once we are awake, we find it more difficult to fall back to sleep. Our sleep is further compromised as we get older because as we age, there are more things to wake us and keep us awake, pain bladder problems, anxiety etc. So, these can cause sleep to be even more disturbed. Because the elderly find it difficult to sleep through the night, they commonly feel the need to nap during the day. However, one consequence of napping during the day may mean that they are further reducing their need for sleep during the night.

With regards to the idea that our ancestors slept in two distinct periods, Ekirch describes many reasons for segmented sleep, e.g., superstition, religion, work, etc. However, he makes little claim of a physiological necessity for this pattern of sleep other than referring to the single study from Wehr.

A simple explanation of segmented sleep is that deep sleep in adults occurs almost exclusively in the first third of the night. Sleep at this time in much less able to be disturbed, and as you know yourself, you rarely wake up in the first 3-4 hours of sleep. Therefore perhaps 'first sleep' merely referred to the first, deep restorative, portion of sleep before we were woken by the need for the toilet, noise, etc.

That's So Me!

So, does any of this information about sleeping touch a chord with you? Have you experienced sleep-deprivation symptoms such as forgetfulness and then worry that early dementia might be just around the corner? Or do you now realise why your partner becomes upset when you happily read late into the night to their dismay and annoyance, and then find you are handed a hasty rebuke in the morning when you can't wake up to get the kids ready or head out for a 6.30 am breakfast with friends?

While it's easy to accept that your soul mate doesn't share your love of pickled herrings or competitive Frisbee, it may not be as easy to accept that this soul mate doesn't share your sleep habits and, worse still wants to sleep apart from you because of your sleep habits. It's a difference many people don't like to think about, let alone talk about, but it's a reality of life that requires recognition and then management.

A 2011 study[62] by Wendy Troxel at the University of Pittsburgh highlighted the importance of considering the interpersonal consequences of sleep and sleep loss. The study found that, among other results, the quality of interactions among married couples is affected by wives' inability to fall asleep at night but not by husbands' sleep problems. Similar results were reported in a 2009 study by the University of Arizona[63] that indicated that on a day-to-day basis, couples' relationship quality affects their sleep, and their sleep also affects their subsequent relationship functioning.

In 1991, Jeffry Larson,[64] a marriage and family therapist at Brigham Young University in Provo, Utah studied 150 couples and found that those couples with mismatched body clocks argued more – 2.13 times per week, compared with 1.6 times per week – and spent less time together in shared activities. They also had less sex too. Larson's recommendations were that couples with differences in their sleep cycles need to accept that body clocks are hardwired, and most people can't re-jig their natural bedtime and waking-up time by more than one hour.

There are many researched and documented differences between the sexes that impact on sleep needs and behaviour. But as each of us is an individual, gender is not the only cause of sleep disturbance. Same-sex couples experience similar incidences of interrupted sleep due to a partner who has different sleep patterns and idiosyncrasies.

The main point to understand is that as humans, we simply don't all have the same needs for sleep. We know men and women are different in so, so many ways, sleeping is just another area that highlights the physiological differences.

In the end, the message from most sleep experts is that you have to accept your hardwiring when it comes to sleep and find the best ways to get the sleep you need to remain healthy. Going to bed two hours later than you would like to, just so you can retire with your partner, is not doing either of you any favours. In fact, the chances are it will have a negative impact on your relationship in the long run.

The final demand to consider about sleep is work in contemporary society. Have you ever wished you could ask your boss if you could start work an hour or two later? If left to wake naturally, would you wake up between 7.30 and 8 am? But the reality of your life means that you need to be up and out the door by about

7.00 am to be at work on time, so you have to resort to it's an alarm clock every morning. This is a common challenge. Western work culture requires most of us to be at work between 8.00, and 9.00 am every day. The construct of the nine to five workday – so eloquently expressed by Dolly Parton – lengthened by increasing travel times created by urban sprawl, sees many people being torn from REM sleep each morning to meet their work requirements. However, for some industries, giving employees the option of arriving at a time that matches their circadian rhythms may not be practically or economically viable.

Then there are shift workers; fly-in fly-out workers; workers in industries that provide night-time services; doctors and nurses in hospitals across the world; and all the other workers such as those who keep the airline industries functioning and have even more irregular and unconventional sleeping timeframes to deal with. Our economic evolution makes all sorts of demands upon us physically, including the need to manage our sleep well enough to work effectively throughout a long day or night. The globalisation of many companies adds an extra dimension to some workers' lives who have to factor in monitoring and interacting with markets in different time zones and catching up with co-workers who have completely different work/sleep lifestyles. This is one of the drivers of an increasingly common complaint about computers and smartphones becoming a 'third person' in beds across the world – an issue we discuss in the next chapter.

Tech Support?

For those who have smartphones and are interested in finding out about their sleep cycles, apps are available that monitor your sleep patterns. The information is interesting in itself, but for those who find they feel groggy on waking and are far more tired than they believe they deserve to be, a scientific point of view would point out that their accuracy in measuring sleep/wake is not particularly good.

So now that we know why we need to sleep, it's time to consider the fraught practice of bed-sharing.

Pause for thought...

- How much sleep do you need to function properly? Have you ever taken the time to notice when you are feeling tired and how much sleep you have, or haven't had?
- Is the amount of sleep you need different from your partner?
- What are your optimal sleeping times? How do these times fit in with demands made on you by your partner, your family, your work?
- Are you a lark or an owl? And what is your partner? And what does this mean for you both?
- Do you prefer one long sleep, or do you wake for a noticeable period during the night where you might watch TV or read a book?
- Have you ever displayed any symptoms of sleep deprivation? (Are you displaying them now?)
- Have you ever thought about and noted the

different sleeping patterns or needs of your partner?

- If there are differences, have you named them or discussed them with your partner?

THREE

The truth about bed-sharing

*'Laugh and the world laughs with you, snore and you sleep
alone.'*

Anthony Burgess[65]

A bed has many uses. It's a place to read, throw your
clothes, watch television, chat on the phone, kiss and
cuddle, have sex, jump up and down, cry and feel sad.
However creatively we may choose to use a bed though,
there's no denying that its primary use is for sleeping. And
as discussed in the last chapter, the somewhat prosaic
activity of sleeping is an essential daily, human activity.
So, inevitably we all retire to the bedroom to get our rest.

If you are part of a couple, heading to the bedroom
each night to sleep may, or may not, fill you with a
sense of calm and restfulness. Not to labour a point, but
falling in love with a person does not guarantee a full
complement of items on the compatibility tick list. The

laws of attraction that send us into the arms of another to mate don't consider a raft of incompatibilities that can bite us after the heady glow of early lust wears off.

The 2012 study by the Central Queensland University mentioned earlier found a partner in your bed is more disruptive to sleep than any other noise. In the survey, 57.6% respondents indicated that they slept with a partner, and, of these, 34.5% indicated that their partner disturbed them while getting into bed. 44% stated that their partner disrupted them by tossing and turning, and 58.5% said that their partner's snoring disturbed their sleep. Over 48% said their partner disturbed them by getting up to go to the bathroom at night; 10.1% reported that their sleep was disturbed by their partner getting up to go to the kitchen; 8.1% of respondents were disturbed by their partner answering phone calls, and 35.9% had been disturbed by a partner getting up to go to work.

A 2022 Australian Sleep Awareness survey found that of the 36% of respondents who reported sleeping alone, half of those had a partner. These separate sleepers cited snoring, noise from CPAP machines, and partner movement as the most common reasons for seeking bedroom solitude.

Yet despite all the potential and known problems that go hand-in-hand with the activity, we keep slipping between the sheets with each other with unfailing optimism.

A Parable

If something is presented as normal human behaviour, then you would expect that:

1. humans will have done it for most of their history
2. it would be ubiquitous across most if not all cultures and
3. it would be natural to do it, i.e., you would not have 'learn' how to do it.

In this regard there is no way that alpine skiing can be considered a normal human behaviour in that it is a relatively modern phenomenon, indulged in by a minority of people and cultures, it takes time to learn, some people are better at it than others, some people who have tried it don't enjoy it, and some people just don't fancy doing it.

Now imagine a scenario where someone told you that skiing was, in fact, the norm for humans. They might claim that if you did it as a child, it would be easier to do it as an adult. They might claim that après ski was an excellent time to share the experiences of the day and to make plans. They might claim the health benefits of the exercise and fresh mountain air and ignore the risk of injuries and falls. They might claim that skiing together will make you a happier couple and be an affirmation of your status as a couple and strengthen your relationship. They may claim that because of this, you will have more sex.

All sound good, doesn't it? But then they would also argue that the only way you can ski is to go down the slope in tandem with you partner regardless of your ability, or own ideas about which run you wish to ski and when. You have to ski down the same slope at the same time never more than a couple of feet from you partner, and because you are so close to each other, it is an ideal time to stop, every once in a while, and engage in sexual activity. And the thing is unless you did this, your relationship was obviously doomed to fail, and you would have fewer opportunities for sex.

This whole scenario would be laughable if it were not precisely the argument that people make for sleeping together.

There are good and bad aspects of bed-sharing. The critical determinant is the needs and wants of each individual and how determined that individual is to have those needs and wants to be met. Bedtime behaviours are in themselves mundane. But add in the human elements of temperament, emotion, power plays, relationship dynamics, traditions, morals, pride, changing attitudes, physical health and personality and a set of mundane behaviours can go from being banal to a battlefield.

As discussed, there is the expectation of couples (especially in most Western cultures) who marry or choose to live together that part of the deal of sharing your life with each other includes sharing a bed.

You are a married couple; you are a partnership and sleeping together is a symbol of that.
Amelia, 41, mother of two, married 12 years

It's a social thing that you sleep together; you're in the same room. Loving parents sleep in the same room – not separate rooms.
Anne, 44, senior manager, married 20 years

Think when you find your soulmate you go with the flow – come on you are married share a bed – not difficult. (sic)
Anonymous, www.mamamia.com.au

Being married for the first time at 44 meant it took me a while to adjust to sleeping with someone after a long time of being single and having the whole bed to myself. Despite this, I never considered not sharing a bed – for me, being married meant that as a couple, we would share a bed together.
Sarah, 52, education officer, married 8 years

When my friends came out from the States in the 1990s and built a house with separate rooms, I thought their marriage was over. Word got around our friendship group, and everyone talked about it and thought the same thing.
Von, 72, married 55 years

My emotional side argues that 'It's not normal if you don't sleep next to your husband. You have to make it work' and my logical side screams 'Are you crazy? You need proper sleep! If that means sleeping separately, then so be it!'
Emily, 30, international flight attendant, married 4 years

I think there's something wrong. Her parents aren't sleeping in the same bed anymore.
Gretchen Wieners, Mean Girls

The good stuff

Sharing a bed with another person provides a distinct level of intimacy to a relationship that's hard to replicate. The rituals associated with sharing a space each night, getting ready for bed, spending time alone in the sanctity of a bedroom and lying next to someone – whether you snuggle or barely touch – are part of a relationship without which some couples simply could not live.

> *I find shared sleep deeply sexy; often more so than making love. It's where true love lies, beyond words, beyond sex.*
> Nikki Gemmel, *The Weekend Australian Magazine*, 21-22 January 2012

> *Sharing a bed with my wife Sarah gives me a sense of completeness, togetherness and closeness. As we drift off to sleep together each night, I am reassured that all is well with the world.*
> Thomas, 63, organisational consultant, married 8 years

Physical contact with another human can be calming and comforting and is often sought through sharing a bed and the rhythm of sleep. Many couples speak of the intimacy that bed-sharing brings. This daily act can often be both a personal and public symbol of the closeness a couple shares – usually because sleeping together signifies a closer liaison.

> *I enjoy the intimacy of sleeping with my partner. I sometimes like to cuddle up to her, and she is receptive although she may be asleep. This behaviour is reciprocal. Sometimes we hold hands, sometimes just rest a hand on each other.*
> Chris, 51, builder, with partner for 3 years

> *I love ending the day next to my husband. No matter*

*what's happened in the day ... our bed is our haven
when there's just the two of us. We can share the
day, plan the next day, console and cajole. We can
be tender and touch or fall asleep from exhaustion
with very little said but with the knowledge that we
share the bed, an arm's length away and tomorrow
another day.*

Alana, 60, personal assistant, married 32 years

There is a social aspect to bed-sharing that many couples
enjoy and choose to prioritise over disrupted sleep. In
fact, some may view sleeping with another person – be
it a partner, child, or friend – as a social event in itself. Of
course, many people simply like sharing a bed with their
partner. The cuddling and chatting, and camaraderie
of hopping into this small comfy space each night has
a romantic allure and can be wonderful to share with
another.

Retiring to bed each night can provide the
opportunity to spend quiet time together to debrief on
the day, discuss topics you may not want to bring up in
front of children, have a serious conversation with your
partner on a personal issue, or lie quietly next to each
other in that comfortable silence couples develop over
time and a life shared together. In an increasingly busy
lifestyle, this may be the only time when couples find
the time to be alone with the other to meet a myriad of
needs.

*My wife and I are so busy in our lives that sleeping
together is often the only place we can spend time
alone together. Just knowing that I can at least touch*

her hand and lie next to her is all I need to reconnect each day. I couldn't live without it.
Tony, 47, IT consultancy business development manager, married 25 years

I cherish my time in bed with my partner. I love our little chats before we fall asleep. I love his snuggles in the middle of the night. To the point where I can't sleep if he's not in bed with me.
Trina, www.mamamia.com.au

The one thing I look forward to at the end of each day is the brief moment before we go to sleep when I get to lay my head on my husband's chest and hear his heart beating. We don't talk. But just that brief connection means so much to me. Sleeping together gives us the chance for regular intimacy such as midnight discussions about topics that worry us. Sometimes you can talk about things so much easier when lying next to one another in the dark. Quite often we will hold hands while we are talking about things that worry us and this is reassuring.
Cass, www.villainouscompany.com

Sleeping with another person may also be a habitual activity. Individuals who slept with siblings in a bed or a room as they were growing up may equate safety and security with having another person in close proximity during sleep. There is a gender ideology that women need the protection of men, and this protection may extend to bed-sharing.

I actually sleep *better* with my partner in the bed. I don't think he makes a physical difference, but there's something comforting about him being there. I find it really hard to sleep by myself now if I'm staying at my parents' or overnight at a party. I almost never wake up refreshed if I've slept alone.
Shannon, www.mamamia.com.au

I always go to bed well before my partner, so I fall asleep fine by myself, but if he's away and I know he's not coming to bed that night, I can't get to sleep at all! I have to have the TV on in the other room; I hate sleeping when there's no-one else in the house.
Alena, www.mamamia.com.au

Paul Rosenblatt, author of *Two in Bed: The Social System of Couple Bed Sharing*,[66] says that the cited benefits of sleeping with another are either person-focused, such as warmth, sense of safety and companionship, or couple-focused, such as intimacy, shared experiences and reaffirming the couple's commitment. For those individuals who need a sense of safety security and companionship, sharing a bed can provide this and create an environment conducive to a good night's rest.

So, while there is much that is good, even great, about sleeping with another, there are aspects of the practice that leave a lot to be desired. As sleeping is such a fundamental human need, honestly examining the unpleasant realities of sleep is as vital as enjoying the upside.

The bad stuff

> *"There is not in my opinion anything in nature which*
> *is more immediately calculated totally to subvert*
> *health, strength, love, esteem, and indeed everything*
> *that is desirable in the married state, than that*
> *odious, most indelicate, and most hurtful custom of*
> *man and wife continually pigging[1] together, in one*
> *and the same bed. Nothing is more unwise-nothing*
> *more indecent –nothing more unnatural, than for a*
> *man and woman to sleep, and snore, and steam, and*
> *do everything else that's indelicate together, three*
> *hundred and sixty-five times –every year"*
> 'Dr.' James Graham 1785

Being in close physical contact with any person, in any
setting, for an extended period inevitably creates issues.
Lying next to the same person night after night can be a
breeding ground for all that can be unpleasant between
two people. And while there are behaviours and habits
our partners have that we can learn to live with, such
as leaving the lid off the sauce bottle, or not making the
bed first thing in the morning, a 1999 study by the Mayo
Clinic found that people don't automatically adjust to
sleep disturbances.[67]

Even though Paul Rosenblatt encourages couples
to learn to sleep together, he notes the following about
sharing a bed: "Sleeping together is an achievement of
coordination on many dimensions – where to locate one's
head, body, arms and legs, where to put one's pillow,

---

1   pigging: OED, from the verb 'to pig' meaning "to huddle, live, or sleep
together, esp. in a crowded or disorderly way or in dirty conditions".

how to relate to the blankets, when to talk and not talk, when to touch the other and when not, how to touch the other, what ways of expressing displeasure with the other are acceptable and work, how free one is to toss and turn, what to do when the other makes noise, what to do and not do if one awakens during the night."[68]

It all sounds like such hard work, doesn't it?

And while each couple faces their own proximity issues, there do appear to be some clear winners in the litany of complaints from bed sharers. We're going to look at the 'bad' parts of bed sharing in two categories. First, there are the actual *in-bed* bed behaviours, and then there are the habits and behaviours *around* going to bed.

While these behaviours that can disrupt one partner's ability to sleep, there may also be hidden or more serious medical issues. One person's bed-time annoyance could, in reality, be another's life-threatening medical condition. Throughout the chapter, we will provide information about medical conditions that might lie behind your partner's night-time behaviours and offer some possible solutions that might be of help to you both.

Snoring

Snoring is by far the most common reason why one partner will disturb the other's sleep. And, sorry guys, but it does tend to be men who are most guilty on this charge. The National Sleep Foundation of America supports this stain on your good characters.

Persons most at risk are males and those who

are overweight, but snoring is a problem of both genders, although it is possible that women do not present with this complaint as frequently as men.

The physical and medical reasons for snoring are complex and varied. They range from having one too many alcoholic drinks to life-threatening conditions such as sleep apnoea. So, whether it's the man or the woman snoring in bed, it's a prevalent problem, and it keeps a lot of people awake. Snoring also becomes more frequent and louder as we age. And that's for both men and women. So, if you are smugly reading this and have not yet reached your forties – it's all ahead of you.

I hated my husband because of his snoring. I hated that he could keep me awake and not even know he was doing it. When I would kick him and say 'Please stop snoring' he would say, 'I'm not snoring – what are you talking about?' and then it would be my problem, and I would be furious with him. We could not have stayed in the same bed together because I really resented him for it. I resented the way he reacted. He didn't wake up and say 'I'm really sorry keeping you awake' he would wake up and say 'Stop kicking me – why are you kicking me?' and then resent me.
Frances, 40, mother of 3, married 10 years

When my husband snores I want to say 'go away you sound like a troll'. I think snoring is one of the most unattractive things a person can do. To me, it's a hideous sound, and there's nothing appealing about

someone who snores. So if I can't hear his snoring, he looks much nicer and much more appealing to me.
Rebecca, 47, counsellor, married 20 years

My snoring simply became an issue for us. John tried earplugs, but he couldn't wear them for more than three nights in a row, and I felt bad that he had to.
May, 66, retired, married 40 years

I sleep in a separate room from my partner of more than 20 years because of his snoring. We downloaded an app that measures decibels, and his snoring was at the same sound level as a food processor makes grinding nuts!
Anonymous, www.mamamia.com.au

My father's snoring eventually ended our family holidays in caravans. My brother and I would be up in the annexe at 2 am playing cards because Dad's snoring was as loud as a train.
Kate, 46, lawyer, married 12 years

My mother is renowned for her snoring. To the point where I can only describe it as a whipper snipper next to you! And she snores no matter what, front, back and sides! My father's only saving grace is he falls asleep really quickly and easily, so it's usually not a problem.
Trina, www.mamamia.com.au

Unfortunately, snoring is something over which we have little control. While intermittent snoring can be controlled through fewer beers or wines, for many people, it is embarrassing and a source of frustration. It is a pity that unintended behaviour can have such a significant impact on so many couple's lives. It is genuinely mystifying that some people tell of years of no sleep due to a snoring partner, and yet they have done nothing to address the situation and continue to complain of no sleep.

While your partner may only emit a gentle purr that disturbs you occasionally, the voracity with which some people snore can be quite alarming. The average snorer emits a noise level of 50 decibels. This is equivalent to the noise generated by a normal conversation at home or a large electrical transformer 100 feet away.[69] The Guinness Book of Records[70] reports Koere Walkert from Sweden as one of the loudest snorers. Measured at 93 decibels on 24 May 1993, his snoring is as loud as a belt sander. However, Walkert is a lightweight compared to Jennifer Chapman in Britain, who was recorded snoring at 111.6 decibels at a snoring boot camp in 2009.[71] This puts her as just a little louder than a chain saw, not quite as loud as a hammer drill, but still 8 decibels louder than a low-flying jet.[72]

As a guide,[73] anything over 70 decibels is when your hearing can start to be damaged – so spare a thought for Jennifer Chapman's husband. Sensibly though, he does often sleep in another room, with both bedroom doors shut and sometimes with his head under a pillow.

And fortunately for Jennifer, she wasn't married to John Wesley Hardin. An outlaw who lived in America in the late 1800s, Hardin reportedly shot a sleeping stranger in the room next to him because his snoring was keeping Hardin awake.[74] While many of us may have thought of such extreme action as well, fortunately for thousands of snorting and snuffling partners, we have exercised far greater restraint.

Sleep Apnoea

We have all heard or told stories that involve great feats of snoring that are the cause of disturbed sleep. Although people who snore loudly are frequently the target of bad jokes and the occasional victims of middle-of-the-night elbow thrusts, snoring is no laughing matter. Loud snoring can be a sign that something is seriously wrong with your breathing during sleep. Snoring is a sign that the airway is not fully open and the distinctive sound of snoring comes from efforts to force air through the narrowed passageway.

It is estimated that 10-30% of adults snore. For most sufferers, snoring has no serious medical consequences. But for an estimated 5% of people—often overweight middle-aged men—extremely loud, habitual snoring can be the first sign of a potentially severe disorder—Obstructive Sleep Apnoea (OSA). OSA has a particular pattern of breathing during the night with pauses in the snoring followed by gasps as the breathing starts again. These pauses can last from a few seconds to over a minute and can occur hundreds of times a night. People who have OSA don't breathe properly during sleep; therefore, they do not get enough oxygen. Patients with OSA can have very disturbed sleep often without knowing it; all they may know is that they feel very sleepy during the day.

OSA can seriously disturb sleep producing extreme levels of sleepiness during the day interfering with work and personal life. People with OSA may have trouble concentrating and can become unusually forgetful, irritable, anxious, or depressed. These problems can appear suddenly or can emerge gradually over time. If these problems develop over time, it is common for sufferers to ascribe the sleepiness during the day to the consequences of normal ageing. Because OSA puts a strain on the body, it can trigger high blood pressure, heart failure, heart attacks and stroke and has been linked to a significantly increased risk of car accidents due to the daytime sleepiness.

Often people with OSA seek help for disturbed sleep not realising that OSA may be to blame. People with OSA may notice that they are frequently waking during the night, gasping for air, and thrashing about in their sleep. Because they are often not aware of what is happening during the night, which is why information from the bed partner is so all-important. Sufferers may also complain of morning headaches, and loss of interest in sex and men may experience erectile failure. OSA is most often found in middle-aged men, but anyone can suffer OSA— even children.

It is imperative to seek medical advice if you or your bed partner suspect either of you suffers from OSA. There is good news; however, in that OSA can usually be effectively treated. If you have mild sleep apnoea treatment may include advice on lifestyle management, including helping people lose weight, stop smoking and/or decrease alcohol consumption. Severe OSA is routinely treated with a device known as CPAP

(Continuous Positive Airway Pressure). Other treatments, such as mandibular positioning devices are also available and are useful for some patients. You should consult your GP about the available options.

Movement

Movement in bed can range from innocent repositioning for comfort, through to restless leg syndrome and flailing limbs that can turn the bed into a nightly replay of a good old-fashioned gladiator epic. Some people find they have partnered with a 'floundering whale' who flops around the bed all night, taking the sheets and blankets with them, oblivious to the innocent soul shivering on the other side, fuming quietly or whimpering sadly.

The reality is that sleeping involves movement, especially during the light sleep stages. We all change sleeping position around 20 times a night[75] but Professor Jim Horne, director of Loughborough University's Sleep Research Centre, notes that men seem to shift around more than women.[76] In an experiment conducted at the centre, movement sensors placed on men and women found that men move around twice as much in the night. This fact may help settle some arguments about bedclothes that go awry on a nightly basis.

And while innocent and simple movement might just be annoying, sharing a bed with a 'human windmill' can be life-threatening. There are documented cases of women who have bruised breasts from being rolled on during sleep. Ouch!

I like a lot of personal space. I like to sleep in different positions. On my back, on my tummy, arms behind my head, arms to my side, arms straight up like a soldier (rarely, but I like to keep my options open), legs splayed, knees drawn up to my chest, hanging from the chandelier wearing bunny ears and a tail (okay, so that one is my husband's fantasy). I don't like to be restricted in my movements by anyone pushing my limbs out of the way when I fancy a good stretch.

Kerri, 44, author and blogger, with husband 20 years

My husband and I regularly, accidentally punch or elbow each other in the face at night. We have a queen size, but I think we need to upsize to avoid injury.

littlemisschloe, www.mamamia.com.au

Where do I begin? I have been elbowed and kicked more times than I can remember, had his arm 'thud' on me as he turns over, and pushed with such force that I am jolted out of sleep with such a startle I find it hard to get back to sleep sometimes. I know he doesn't mean to do it and is always apologetic, but I often wonder if it would be a legal reason to justifiably let me hurt him.

Chloe, 32, accountant

While having someone kicking, punching, tossing, and turning in your bed may be very annoying and disturbing to your sleep, Meadows et al. found that about one-third of objectively measured nocturnal awakenings were common to both bed-partners – effectively meaning that one or other of the bed partners was waking the other when they themselves woke. There could be several explanations for movements during the night most of them are natural and normal however some can be serious medical problems.

Periodic Limb Movement Disorder (PLMD)

PLMD is a sleep disorder where the sufferer repeatedly makes kicking and jerking movements with their legs or arms during sleep, usually without being aware of it. As the sufferer is unaware, they are doing it, the bed partner is the one to notice this behaviour. The repeated movements can disturb the sufferer's sleep, and similarly to sleep apnoea; they may notice that they are suffering from daytime sleepiness for no apparent reason. Women are more likely to suffer from the condition than men and causes can include too much caffeine, stress, and other mental health problems so if your partner repeatedly jerks their limbs during the night or indeed frequently seems to punch or kick you then you should investigate PLMD.

Restless Legs Syndrome (RLS)

RLS is a neurological movement disorder involving unpleasant feelings occurring in the legs and described as painful, tingling, itching, or prickling. Because these unpleasant feelings occur at rest and are relieved by movement, RLS sufferers have difficulty sleeping. Approximately 5-10% of the population is affected, although it is twice as common in females as in males. About 80% of those with RLS also have PLMD (see above). Deficiencies in substances, especially iron, are likely to play a role in RLS. RLS is extremely common in pregnancy, particularly during the 3rd trimester. Iron and/ or vitamin B12 supplements have been found to be helpful in reducing RLS as is having cold/warm compresses and massage. Also, as with most other sleep problems, avoiding caffeine, nicotine, and alcohol can help.

Sleepwalking

Sleepwalking, aka somnambulism, is a general term used to describe disorders where people perform simple behaviours during their sleep. These can range from simply sitting up and looking around, to walking around and performing tasks usually done while awake, e.g., going to the fridge for a drink of milk, going to post a letter or even getting in a car and driving. Somnambulism occurs during deep Slow Wave Sleep (SWS) sleep.

Sleep is not an 'all or nothing' phenomena. Parts of your brain can be asleep while others are awake. This means that if during deep sleep a particular part of the brain wakes up—partial arousal—then it is possible to carry out behaviour for which that part of the brain is responsible for, e.g., walking, talking, etc., without being conscious of it, because the conscious part of the brain is still asleep.

Sleepwalking is reported to occur in approximately one or two per cent of adults. There is a strong genetic link in the occurrence of sleepwalking, but other causes can include over-tiredness, stress, sleeping pills, alcohol – essentially anything that fragments sleep can precipitate these partial arousals. Adopting a regular bedtime and avoiding things that can disturb sleep help, but it is also essential to make the environment as safe as possible. Because sleepwalking occurs during deep sleep, it is most liable to occur in the first third of the night in adults.

Sleep Sex

Sleep sex — or sexsomnia — is a parasomnia that can occur during deep sleep and involves a person engaging in sexual activities (including penetration) while still asleep. In extreme cases, sexsomnia has been alleged as the cause of instances of sexual assault, including rape. Sexsomniacs do not remember the acts that they perform while they are asleep. Sexsomnia can co-occur alongside other sleep disorders such as sleepwalking, sleep apnoea, night terrors and bedwetting. It can be triggered by stress, previous sleep deprivation, and excessive consumption of alcohol or drugs. Such 'extreme' behaviour is, of course, going to disturb the bed partner but perhaps, more importantly, it is probably going to be hard for the bed partner to understand the fact that this behaviour is not intentional.

REM Behaviour Disorder

REM behaviour disorder is a condition that is often confused with sleepwalking. As its name suggests, REM behaviour disorder occurs during REM sleep, not SWS like sleepwalking. Usually, during REM sleep, we lose muscle tone so that we cannot act out our dreams as such we are effectively, temporarily, paralysed. However, in some people, this paralysis does not occur, and therefore they can physically act out their dreams. REM behaviour disorder can occur because of drugs of abuse, medicines or alcohol or in people withdrawing from them. It can also be a precursor of Parkinson's disease and is common in dementia. Also, there is a tiny population of otherwise normal older men who seem to become chronic sufferers.

Menstrual Cycle and Sleep

For women, the hormones oestrogen and progesterone that play a role in regulating the menstrual cycle can also influence sleep and circadian rhythms. Many women report 2–3 days of disrupted sleep during each cycle with an increased number of awakenings and other sleep disturbances during their premenstrual period. This leads to an increase in restlessness and thus increased fidgeting, which can disturb a partner's sleep. Oral contraceptives affect body temperature regulation, and this can affect sleep. Women on oral contraceptives have more stage 2 sleep and less of the restful and restorative deep sleep.

Pregnancy and Sleep

Sleep is disrupted substantially during pregnancy and postpartum, with a prevalence of insomnia ranging from 15% to 80%. After conception, most women report daytime fatigue and the need for longer night-time sleep. From the second trimester onwards, the time spent asleep begins to decrease and sleep quality becomes poor. During the second and third trimesters, nocturnal awakenings, fatigue, leg cramps, difficulty in sleeping in certain positions and shortness of breath become more common. Pregnant women, particularly during the final trimester, have a heightened risk of snoring, sleep apnoea and restless legs syndrome.

Menopause

Menopausal women often experience hot flashes during the night that can disrupt sleep. Ninety per cent of women experience these symptoms with 25-50% describing sleep disturbances. Hot flashes and night sweats can cause repeated awakenings because of the sensation of heat and sweating as well as increased heart rate and anxiety. Because the sleep disturbance is related to temperature, it is important for sleep to have a cool temperature in your bedroom with light, cotton, bed linen and you want to avoid anything that also raises body temperature before bed.

Night-time comfort breaks

Another everyday movement during the night is one partner getting up to go to the toilet. The increase of ensuite bathrooms in modern houses means that not only is there disruption from the act of getting out of bed; there can also be some disturbingly audible proof of the activity.

For men sharing a bed with a pregnant woman, frequent toilet trips during the night – while good training for the sleeplessness to come – can be equally as disturbing.

> *While I understand that my husband needs to go to the toilet during the night, must the activity involve the broken waterfall effect, a couple of farts and that much sighing? It's always been a bone of contention between us. He won't even shut the door – 'it takes too much time'.*
> Sue, 48, married 12 years

> *I know it's wrong to be angry about things related to pregnancy, but my wife would go to the toilet about 5–6 times a night in the last couple of months of her pregnancy. I was too frightened to tell her that it was really disturbing my sleep. I just drank a lot of coffee at work. It wasn't a great time.*
> Simon, 43, IT manager

> *About 6 months into my pregnancy, I just moved out into the other room. That way I could spread out, toss and turn and go to the toilet as many times as I needed.*
> daisy123, www.mamamia.com.au

Nocturia

One of the leading causes of sleep impairment as we get older, besides those associated with natural ageing, is nocturia, i.e., needing to go to the bathroom multiple times during the night. More than one bathroom visits a night is considered a problem, and the more often you get up to go to the bathroom, the more disturbed your sleep will be. The frequent nocturnal awakenings and the resultant sleep disturbance associated with nocturia can result in a severe disruption of sleep, leading to daytime fatigue and sleepiness together with a decrease in cognitive functioning and alertness.

Rates of nocturia increase with age. So, while 10% of the general population over 20 years has nocturia two or more times per night, in the 50-59 age group, 58% of men and 66% of women experience nocturia. It is also important to note that while the sleep disturbance of the person with nocturia is of primary importance, it should also be remembered that the sleep of the bed partner can also be significantly disturbed by nocturia, which unlike many other sleep disorders actually requires the sufferer to get out of bed.

Temperature

The different preferences in sleeping temperature are another way to heat things up in the bedroom, whether talking about bed coverings, breezes through an open window or air conditioning.

Research suggests that men don't perceive temperature as sensitively as women, which is why they feel warmer. One theory is that women tend to have more blood circulating their core organs, and less around their extremities, such as their hands and feet, which are the body's temperature sensors.

Hands up, those ladies who have slipped their cold

feet or hands on to body parts of their male partner to warm them? Jennifer knows that she will hear the loud protests of her husband when she slips into her husband's bed for a cuddle before heading to her bed for the night. Similarly, hands up, anyone who hates it when your partner tries to suck the warmth from you with their cold hands or feet? And if we are really being honest… who hasn't had a bit of a giggle when angling your cold bottom into your partner's warm embrace for a quick spoon before you slip off to sleep? Yes, it's all good fun, until one of you feels that you are being used as a human water bottle.

Typically, women prefer their sleeping environment to be warmer than men. This is backed up by Paul Rosenblatt's research; he found that 75% of the heterosexual couples he interviewed reported that when one of them was warmer than the other, it was usually the man. But not always. A woman can be the partner generating the most heat. Research has shown that women's body temperature rises by as much as one degree towards the end of their menstrual cycle.[77] Hormonal changes during pregnancy and menopause can also lead to a raised temperature.

My husband and I have had trouble sleeping together. I tend to sleep 'hot' and prefer a thinner blanket, while he sleeps 'cold' and likes a giant quilt. It took two and a half years, but we realised along the way that instead of a nightly debate over whose favourite blanket we would use, we would each cram our own onto the bed. We no longer have the 'your blanket makes me too hot/cold' discussion in the morning.
Kate, www.mamamia.com.au

My wife requires more warmth in the bed. She needs a quilt most nights to sleep under, but I want to toss it off. Each person requires their own comfort level.
Bruce, 68, married 3 years

I was undergoing chemotherapy and radiation and became impossible to sleep with. My changes in body temperature became a big issue for us both and part of the raft of reasons we moved to separate beds.
Brooke, 52, education professional, married 30 years

My husband likes to be very scientific about things. So when I reach for an extra blanket, wriggle my icy feet and complain 'it's cold …' he'll look at the thermometer he has nearby for just such occasions and tell me that it's not cold, because it's 20 degrees in the bedroom. Different people just feel the cold differently. I can see that from my kids – one cocooned under a mound of blankets, the other spreadeagled on top of the sheets. When you are sharing a bed though, that can be tricky. I have surrendered any notion of enjoying an electric blanket. He tolerates the quilt in winter, so long as most of the feathers have been distributed away from him. Little by little, we have reached an accommodation about the arrangement of blankets – and the desirability of bed socks – even though I know we will never agree on whether it is 'cold'.
Kate, 46, lawyer, married 12 years

Bedroom temperature can play a significant role in ensuring good sleep. In general, the bedroom should be cool. This is because during the night your body temperature naturally drops; thus, the body needs to lose heat, and this is done mainly through the head and face as these are the only bits that usually stick out from under the duvet. Thus, a cool bedroom facilitates this heat loss, (Interesting historical fact – as bedrooms have become warmer, so the wearing of a nightcap has disappeared!).

So how cool is cool? Well, many experts say that the ideal temperature for the bedroom is approximately 16-18ºC (60-65ºF), although this is a matter of personal preference. However, while a cool bedroom is essential, it is also important that the temperature in your direct sleeping environment, i.e., under the duvet, is comfortable. This temperature should be close to a thermo-neutral temperature (i.e., approx. 29ºC). Usually, you can heat your 'sleeping space', to the correct level solely with the body heat you generate during the night but if the bed is unusually cold, a hot water bottle can help get the temperature to a comfortable level.

If the room is too hot, or you are too hot under the duvet, it is more difficult for the body to lose the body heat that it needs to, and this will cause disturbed sleep. (Note that this is the reason why alcohol and big meals should be avoided too close to bedtime, as they are both highly calorific the body has to burn off these calories, this generates heat, and thus the body needs to shift this extra heat additionally). Poor sleep can also result if you are too cold in bed either because the room is too cold, so you lose too much body heat, or the bed is too cold so that it is hard for the body to achieve its optimal temperature for sleep (a hot water bottle, bed socks or even wearing a nightcap can help).

Getting your bed partner can complicate achieving the right temperature as they may need a different combination from you to achieve their comfortable sleep temperature. This is particularly important for women because of the hormonal fluctuations they experience through life interfere with their ability to lose body temperature, and this can make their sleep more disturbed and increase restlessness during the night. Using two single duvets on a double bed maybe a way around this or there are some duvets available that have a different tog rating on one side than on the other.

The correct temperature in the bed and bedroom is vital for good sleep and involves the right combination of air temperature, duvets, bedclothes, etc., to hopefully achieve the correct result for you.

Breathing

Whether we are asleep or awake, respiration just keeps on happening. Like snoring, this is an uncontrollable behaviour as we don't know that our mouth falls open after we fall asleep. However, as the wee hours of the morning approach, the wafting smell or the raspy sound of a loved one's breath is less than welcome.

After 15 years and three kids together a queen bed just doesn't cut it, when it is time to sleep, I need my space! I have to face away from my hubby while sleeping; I hate being breathed on! I have actually said to my hubby that things would be a lot better if he didn't breathe overnight! Daytime breathing only!
Sarah, www.mamamia.com.au

I hate, hate, hate being breathed on! I tell Mr W he is
like a dragon breathing on my neck and the sound is
like a plane taking off in my ear!
Whippersnapper, www.mamamia.com.au

A king-sized bed has made the sleeping experience
better. In our queen-sized bed, I always woke up with
a cricked neck from sleeping facing away from him
as I hate being breathed on in the night.
Anonymous, www.mamamia.com.au

Like snoring, poking and prodding might make the problem of a partner breathing in your direction stop, but just like snoring, for how long? We do wonder if Darth Vader ever shared a bed with a partner.

Children and pets

Those who follow through on the laws of attractions and produce children often face additional demands on their bed real estate. Not only do you have to share with your loved one, but you may also have to share your minimal and prized space with some little loved ones as well.

For some, bed space may progress from a small crib to a bigger cot, to a single bed, to a double or queen bed – all by yourself. Then you start sleeping with your partner, and your bed space is halved, then the children come along, and you find yourself gripping on for dear life to the last foot of space at the edge of the mattress as the toenails of your toddler rake your calves.

The balancing act of trying to allow everyone in a

family to get enough sleep often forces the hand of many parents who give in and let children share their bed.

> *After years of bed-hopping to accommodate our two children who would not spend a full night in their own bed, we gave in and just started sleeping with one child in our bed and one of us in the spare bed in their room. It's been close to 10 years now, and even after recently paying them $5 a night to sleep in their own bed, after about four weeks, the eldest boy started coming through to our room again, so we are back to sleeping apart.*
> Michael and Liza, 41 and 39, married 10 years

> *My partner and I have been together 8 years and slept in separate rooms for about 3 years now. I used to and probably still would love sleeping with him, but since we have had kids, 2 boys within 15 months that both co-sleep, I've shifted to the spare room. We have a king-sized bed, but I was still constantly annoyed and as a result, waking up shirty too. He loves the kids in the bed, and it honestly doesn't bother him if he is woken up by a foot in the face or a cry for a cup of milk. I used to feel guilty, but now I don't, I realise sometimes you gotta do what you gotta do!*
> Lola, www.mamamia.com

The one positive aspect of this shared-sleeping problem is that it has an endpoint. Most parents can be confident that they won't have to co-sleep with or make room in their bed for, their teenager. At least, one hopes not.

Some people could easily substitute 'pet' for 'child'. In fact, we'll bet there are some who have done it already. Some of us are more than happy to share our beds each night with a furry creature, but others think that any animal in the bed is a non-negotiable 'no'.

So, what happens when you meet your soul mate, and the whirlwind romance leads you to the bedroom to find that Fluffy gets to sleep in the middle of the bed, and then at the bottom, and later in the middle again, and then back to the bottom each night? Because humans can become terribly attached to their animals, this issue can be as significant as the arguments for or against children sleeping in bed.

One reason why, for most of human history, men and women have not shared a bed is the fact that for most of this time, the accepted norm was for mothers to sleep with their babies. And given the number of children women had in the past, this probably meant most of their married life. This practice is still prevalent in much of the world, including countries like Japan and India. By sleeping next to its mother, an infant receives protection, warmth, emotional reassurance, and is easily feed. However, recently in Western societies, the practice of mothers and infants sleeping together has been actively discouraged. While this is not the place to thoroughly rehearse the arguments for and against co-sleeping it should be noted that Western parents are taught that they should not co-sleep with their child, and two reasons cited for this advice are that:

1. it will make the infant too dependent on them
2. open up the risk of accidental suffocation or Sudden Infant Death Syndrome (SIDS).

On the issue of a child becoming too dependent on their mother the, albeit few, psychological studies done in this area suggest that children who have 'co-slept' in a loving and safe environment become better-adjusted adults than those who were encouraged to sleep without parental contact or reassurance.

One of the findings of Klösch et al. was objectively "…that women are more disturbed by the male presence in bed than the man by a woman's presence" and that this may be due to that fact that "women appear to react more to the presence of another individual in bed. This may be a logical consequence of the maternal role in infant sleep and development". From an evolutionary point of view and throughout history, and still, in most cultures, it is the woman's role to sleep with the baby to monitor the baby through the night. However, because we have recently replaced this very natural way of sleeping with 'couple sleeping' the woman is still functioning in her evolutionary 'mother mode' of monitoring the person in bed with them.

So, in simple terms, women have poorer sleep than men when they co-sleep because women are essentially reacting to the man in the bed in the same way she would do to an infant monitoring their breathing and their movements to ensure that nothing is wrong. Basically, our society has replaced the infant in the mother's bed with the partner who in this respect is just a huge baby.

There were gender differences in the perceived causes of sleep problems; women are more likely than men to perceive children and pets and partners as causes of their sleep problems.[78]

It should be remembered that cats and dogs can

snore just like humans. And although dogs can and will adapt to their owner's sleeping habits and positions, cats cannot, or more probably will not, give up their lifestyle and will sleep wherever they feel comfortable — however much that may disturb you. In a survey only presented as a porter, but often referred to in the media, Dr John Shepard,[79] the Mayo Clinic in the USA, asked 300 patients seeking help for sleep disorders about their pets and sleep. He found that 53% of pet owners considered that their sleep was disrupted by their pet to some extent every night. However, only 1% felt their sleep was disrupted for more than 20 minutes a night on average.

To cuddle or not to cuddle

Is your idea of sleeping heaven when your partner takes you in their arms and holds you tight through the night until dawn's rays slip through the curtains the next morning? Or does this scenario fill with you dread, make your hands shake wildly at your side, and make you feel icky and want to say 'ewwwww'?

Just like we have different tolerance levels about activities such as holding hands and cuddling and kissing in public, some of us don't want to be held in a loving embrace all night. Because men generally fall asleep faster, women can be left trapped under a well-meaning but vice-like arm. There is also the problem of ongoing physical contact creating sweaty bodies that are neither pleasant to feel or smell nor great for the sheets.

Spooning your loved one as you succumb to blissful

slumber makes for a great visual in the movies but doesn't really accommodate the human need for changing positions as we cycle through our sleep patterns every night.

I'm at the start of the trying to convince a newish boyfriend that sleeping separately is okay. Yes, I love the snuggling and the cuddling, but when it's time to sleep I really dislike being touched. I'm a light sleeper and have rheumatoid arthritis, so it's hard for me to get comfortable enough to sleep well at the best of times. Having a boyfriend who feels the constant need to be touching me somehow rather complicates things. It's a really hard topic to discuss with him without feeling like I'm being cold or mean!
Em, www.mamamia.com.au

I like to cuddle up to my wife's back as we fall asleep together – I think it's called spooning. After enjoying this for about 5 minutes, I face reality, rollover, and arrange my 3 pillows the way I need them so I can sleep comfortably.
Max, 43, company director, married 18 years

Other in-bed sleeping problems

While one could fill a good portion of this book with what can go wrong when lying in a bed next to another; we'll leave the discussion there and leave you with a list of further complications that can be found between the sheets. The list is not definitive, which is why there are some spaces at the bottom to fill in the ones you think we've missed.

- The size of the bed
- The firmness of the bed
- Who gets to sleep on which side of the bed
- Sheet textures
- Amount and size of pillows
- Different sleep positions
- Teeth grinding
- Sweating
- Getting up in the middle of the night (not just for the toilet)
- Waking from dreams and nightmares
- Going to bed angry
- Sleepwalking
- Sleep talking
- Insomnia
- Illness – temporary or long term
- _____
- _____
- _____

Despite what women say …size does matter

A standard UK double bed is 4 ft 6 ins wide which means you and your bed partner each have 2 ft 3 ins (68.6cm) of space. However, the single bed that you had as a child was either 2 ft 6 ins (76.2cm) or 3ft (91.4cm), which means as an adult you have in essence got either 3 ins (7.6cm) or 9 ins (22.9cm) less space to sleep in than you child. Your child shares their bed with a 'glow in the dark' Teletubby. You, however, share your bed with a kicking, punching, farting, snoring, duvet hugger, and you wonder why you are not sleeping well. So, one of the easiest ways of getting a better night's sleep is to get a bed that's more than 4 ft 6 ins (137.2cm) wide, essentially get a bed as big as you can fit into your bedroom.

As well as nightly tussles when in the bed, there are also the struggles that happen before you even reach the bed or turn out the light.

As outlined in the last chapter, sleeping needs differ from person to person. If you are lucky enough to share similar sleeping needs in regard to getting ready to sleep, the time you go to bed and how long you need to sleep, then well done. However, the reality for many is that they have different bedroom behaviours that can wear down a once happily-shared activity.

Preparing to sleep

Human behaviour is swathed in habit and ritual. Learned behaviours that are replayed consciously or that happen without much thought at all, guide us through each day, week, month, and year. When it comes to going to bed, having a ritual or routine is something that begins when we are babies and don't have the slightest idea of the conditioning to which we are being exposed. Cultural factors vary, but many of you have experienced the practice of children having a set bedtime routine that involves a bath, a story reading and then being tucked into bed nice and early. This traditional approach to our early sleeping behaviour is often the origin of the rituals we adopt as we grow older, which leads me to the first, widespread habit that people have when it comes to going to bed – reading before sleeping.

Similar to snoring, to read or not to read before sleep is an everyday battle fought out in beds across the world. The Big Sleep Survey[80] conducted in 2010 in Australia, with over 12,000 people participating, found that 40% of people like to read when they go to bed, while the Central Queensland University study[81] reported that 59.7% of people like to read in bed. Both results are significant. Reading in bed is a disruptive activity (for the sleeping party) that involves having a light on as well as movement and sound (from the page-turning).

Having a room of one's own was a revelation. First, there was the realisation that I could read as long as I wanted, even with the main light on if I so desired. I've always read in bed – right from the days when I used to hide a flashlight under my pillow so I could continue after my mother had pronounced: 'Lights out.' But during the years of sharing a bed with David, this habit had become one of our great bones of contention: 'Can't you turn off the light? I can't sleep.' Even a specially purchased, tiny light that hooked over the cover of the book was too much for him. He would complain he couldn't sleep, and when I hid it over the edge of the bed, ruining my eyesight in the gloom, he would whine, 'But I can hear you turning the pages!' But then he liked to fall asleep with the radio on, and you can't concentrate on your own novel when Radio 4's 'Book at Bedtime'

is burbling in the background. Now, though, I can do as I please.
Dame Jenni Murray, British journalist and broadcaster for *The Guardian*

My husband is a shift worker, which is an issue. Being an 'owl', I never felt that I could go into my bedroom and feel free to do anything. No activity with noise was allowed, and no reading could happen because there was to be no light in the room. I missed reading in bed.
Anne, 44, senior manager, married 20 years

Neil is a reader, and I can't sleep with the light on. When he would read all night because he couldn't sleep, I would go to the spare room. Now though, he will mostly go to the spare room to read as he needs to, to help him get back to sleep.
Ann, 46, HR professional, married 19 years

As we got older and I became more liberated, I thought why should I have to go to bed when he wants to go and why should I have to turn the lights off when he wants to go to sleep. If I wanted to continue to read, he would complain about the light from my table light keeping him awake.
Von, 72, married 55 years

Watching television in bed is another activity that some find relaxing and soporific, and others find it anything but. A 2009 study[82] of 21,475 adults by the Division of Sleep and Chronobiology at the University of Pennsylvania found that television viewing is the most dominant pre-sleep activity, accounting for almost 50% of pre-bedtime, a statistic which was repeated in the Central Queensland University study. The topic even featured prominently in the movie *Sex in the City 2*: Carrie was most unhappy when Big decided to install a television in the bedroom of their New York apartment.

TV creates light and sound and causes similar problems to reading between couples.

I will never cease to be amazed at how my wife's interest in crappy TV increases in direct proportion to how late at night it is. She will be fighting to stay awake, but intent on getting to the end of another 'Celebrity Something' show no matter what the cost is next morning. The hum of the TV keeps me awake in itself, even without any volume. I will sometimes fall asleep on the couch just to avoid watching the rubbish. It really annoys me, but she insists it helps her sleep. I think it just helps her stay awake.
Wilson, 43, married 15 years

TV had a great bearing on us moving to separate rooms. Margaret had a TV in the bedroom, and I hated it. Absolutely detested it. Why? When I go to bed, I go to bed to sleep. If I want to watch TV, I can do it in the lounge room. When I wanted to go to sleep, Margaret would have to turn the TV off and go out to the lounge room to continue watching her show. And then she would disturb me when she came back to bed.
John, 58, building contractor, married 30 years

*My husband watches TV to wind down and fall
asleep. The problem was that he would lie on the
couch to watch TV, fall asleep, but when he woke up,
turned the TV off and walked down the hall to come
to bed, he would be too awake to fall asleep again.
He just stays on the couch now.*
Suzette, 40, administrative assistant, married 17 years

Then there are those who can't face eight hours of
slumber without nourishment and take a snack to eat
and/or drink when they hop into bed. Despite the risk
of crumbs or drips and drops of food in the bed and on
the bedclothes, an American study found 32% of people
polled take meals and snacks to bed.[83]

*My husband eats in bed, which I cannot stand. He
leaves plates and bowls and water bottles by the
bed. I love lovely linen, and every time I bought new
linen, it would have chocolate ice cream or chocolate
on it, which would never come out. I don't have that
now, because he is eating in his bed, in his room.*
Anne, 44, senior manager, married 20 years

Staying connected

Developments in contemporary living create new
challenges for the modern couple; an array of devices
such as laptops, notebooks, tablets, e-readers, and
smartphones are now a feature of pre-sleep activity.
For some couples, it's not just pre-sleep either, but also
during the night and first thing in the morning. Wireless
networks are commonplace in homes and have given

technology addicts the ability to be online anywhere and anytime.

Almost a third of participants in the 2010 Australian Big Sleep Survey[84] keep a mobile phone in the bedroom at night, with TVs, laptops, iPads, and radios found in roughly 15% of bedrooms. In 2011, Ikea[85] conducted a study of two million people and found that 22% admitted to using a computer in bed (the Central Queensland University study reported 77.9% of respondents said they used a laptop in bed[86]).

Compelling and arguably essential reasons such as checking emails, Facebook and Twitter updates, financial information and sports results are the most common reasons for justifying the need to take a device to bed. And it's not just the fact that your partner is more interested in the screen than you, it's the audible detritus that comes with the electronica.

Salmela, et al[87] found that 13% of people described being disturbed by their partner's use of electronic media in bed. Individual use of smartphones in bed was found to be the normal practice among a majority of participants, being largely used to aid relaxation, and in preparation for sleep.

My husband has headphones listening to music
when I am trying to sleep. I can still hear the music,
and it drives me nuts. (I think it is very anti-social for
him to have headphones in bed!)
Anonymous, www.mamamia.com.au

The iPad is the third person in our relationship.
Morning, noon and night, my partner is emailing

friends, work colleagues and all the other stuff like
Facebook and the web. He knows I don't like the
iPad being used in bed, but thankfully I mostly fall
asleep, and it doesn't disturb me.
Pete, 32, banking professional

Just as books create noise when pages are turned, devices will 'bing' and beep with alerts; click when keyboards are used and throw out a luminous glow that can light up a room just as much as a bedside light. Many of us enjoy being able to sit in bed and use our laptop when needed or watch videos on our iPhone. Our bed partners may be very attached to their iPad using it last thing at night and first thing in the morning.

If this is the area that troubles you most, there is a comprehensive study available that was done by the Sleep Foundation in America in 2011[88] about devices in the bedroom.

There have been numerous studies showing that computer game playing, internet use, television viewing, possession of mobile phones and socialising are linked with reduced sleep, and reduced opportunities for sleep in teenagers,[89] and there is no reason to believe the same is not true of adults.

One of the other problems of technology use is that exposure to artificial light, particularly from LED light, commonly used in TVs, computer screens and handheld electronic devices such as tablets during the evening and at night, can block the effects of brain cells that help promote feelings of sleepiness, as well as suppressing the release of the 'sleep hormone' melatonin. At the same time, artificial light can also stimulate brain cells associated with alertness. This is because LEDs produces a light that is rich in blue and blue-green spectrums, which are the colours that are interpreted by the brain as signifying daytime.

Therefore, using these blue light-rich screens at night will be disruptive to our sleep. So, avoid using technology such as your smartphone, iPad, TV, and laptop at least 45 minutes before your intended hour of retiring.

Light and sound

A dark, quiet room is the gold standard for sleeping. But how quiet is quiet? And how dark is dark? The earlier chapter on the science of sleep touched on the answer for why we prefer a dark environment, but it's a little bit of a 'chicken and egg' question. As melatonin is produced in the body when it gets dark, this means that we tend to sleep when it's dark; and we also need darkness to produce the melatonin to make us sleepy. Prior to the invention of electricity, artificial light didn't confuse our melatonin production, so more people retired to bed earlier. Also, without power, there weren't as many night-time activities anyway, so going to bed was the preferred option for most people.

A recent US study[90] found that sleeping in a room with too much light can cause depression. Scientists that conducted the study found that "even just the glow from leaving the television on while you sleep can be enough to trigger the effect and a lack of darkness during sleeping hours can cause changes to the brain and depressive symptoms". Some people do not like a completely dark room, possibly the result of having a night light as a child, and equally, some cannot bear even a sliver of light disturbing their sleep.

Noise in the bedroom can take many forms. We have already touched on issues such as noise from the turning of a page and sound from electronic devices. However, on the opposite end of the spectrum, there are people who like to have constant noise while they sleep. A commonly sought sound is the constant hum of an air conditioner or a fan. For some, this is more than just a temperature issue; it's that they can't sleep without some type of noise in the bedroom – they cannot 'do' quiet. Our individuality dictates the degrees of dark and quiet; we need to create our optimal sleeping environment.

While not my story, I clearly remember a school friend's sister who slept with clocks in her room. We're not talking a couple: if memory serves, it was over 20. All clocks were ticking clocks, and I was always fascinated by how she could possibly sleep at night. Being a light sleeper, it has been a story that has stayed with me. As she was unmarried at the time I knew her; I used to think about what her husband would say and do when she eventually married. I still do.
Holly, 33, British public servant

I cannot sleep without the fan on in the room. It's not only the feeling of the air moving over my body but the constant hum that it makes. For me, that 'hum' drowns out any other noise that might keep me awake.
Brian, 47, transport worker, married 22 years

How dark is dark?

Light, particularly blue-rich light from the su
computers smartphones, etc., can inhibit the sec
of melatonin, which is a hormone that signals the
that it is time for sleep. Even small amounts of light
from your alarm clock, can be detected through c
eyelids. Therefore, your bedroom needs to be as
as possible, use opaque curtains or blackout blin(
block light from outside, just a few minutes of sur
is necessary to tell your body that it is daytime. In
the room, remove or cover light-producing devices
remember that clocks with red digits are less disrup
than ones with white or blue digits; so, either rep
yours or turn it to face away from you.

The sound of silence

Your bedroom should be as quiet as possible. The Wc
Health Organisation says that overnight the sound le
should be an average of 35dBA with intermittent pea
of 45dBA. It is a simple fact that some noise can distu
sleep, the reason for this is that when you sleep, you a
vulnerable, seemingly unaware of your surrounding
From an evolutionary point of view, this would put yc
at a disadvantage, i.e., something big and hairy can fir
and eat you, so you have to be alert to threats even whi
you are asleep. Because of this, each of us wakes u
hundreds of times during our sleep to check that we ar
still safe and secure.

These awakenings are very short, no more than 1-

seconds, and you are not aware that you have them. If the brain does not detect anything of 'importance' then you can safely go back to sleep, however, if you perceive something in the environment that is not right, e.g., an unexpected noise, your 'primitive' brain needs to be sure that this is not a threat. So, you become fully awake to process and rationalise what is going on. However, you do not wake up to each and every noise, the sound has to be 'meaningful,' i.e., the brain perceives it as important or a threat, for it to disturb your sleep. This means that you can get used to sounds that initially seem very disturbing. This will take at least a couple of weeks as your brain works out that a particular noise is not a threat, and it is safe for you to ignore it.

The fact that you can adapt to some sounds in time does not help when you are staying somewhere temporarily, such as on holiday, so in these situations, it is probably easiest to just carry some earplugs. Of course, if the sound is loud enough regardless of how meaningful it is, it will wake you up, particularly in the latter part of the night when your sleep is naturally lighter and more easily disturbed. Ideally, your bedroom should be as quiet as possible, but this may not be an easy option. If you cannot create a quiet bedroom, then you might want to try using other sounds, e.g., listening to relaxing music or the drone of an electric fan, to distract the brain from the more disruptive noises. It doesn't matter what noise you listen to; the most important thing is that whatever it is your brain does not have to listen to it actively, so your favourite piece of music will probably work best.

Sleep Sanctuary

When at the University of Surrey, Neil designed the finest bedrooms ever constructed for sleep. They were incredibly quiet, temperature-controlled and when you put the lights out, they were very, very dark, (the other key points were a single bed and a teddy bear!). The construction of the bedrooms was a brick-built outer room an inner suspended room consisting of 10cms of acoustic foam and 10cms of acoustic tiling which gave a room-to-room sound attenuation of approximately 85 decibels. This essentially meant that the world's loudest snorer could sleep in the room next door and their snoring would not be loud enough to wake you up. So, although these rooms were pretty much the ideal sleeping environment, they are also probably everything that your bedroom at home is not.

The first important thing to remember is that your bedroom should be the room devoted to sleep. It is the 'bed' room, not the office, games room, gym, or cinema, or even your sex dungeon but the place for sleep. Some languages, such as German 'schlafzimmer' and Dutch 'slaapkamer', make this explicit it is the 'sleep room'. Therefore, everything about the room should be devoted to the optimising of sleep, and thus as discussed elsewhere, it should be cool, quiet, dark, and comfortable. But more than that it should be a sanctuary from the stresses and strains of the world, a place where you can feel safe and secure, a retreat from daytime life.

Up and go

How do you like to be woken in the morning? By a pair of twittering bluebirds gently rousing you from your night of slumber with their songs? Or by the shattering blast of a hard rock radio station so that you know for sure you are going to stay awake? Are you a serial snoozer who must hit that button for another 10 minutes of sleep so many times that you struggle to catch the bus each day? Or are you a lark who went to bed so early that dawn's first light woke you and allowed you to pop out for a quick half-hour run before most of us even realised it was day?

How we are woken can impact on our mood and attitude right from the second we open our eyes. As noted, being woken at the wrong time in your sleep cycle can leave you feeling out of sorts and struggling to get your eyes open and find your nice inner person. If you've ever been accused of 'getting out of bed on the wrong side', it could be attributed to when you were woken rather than where you were in bed.

If a couple retires to bed at different times, but wake at the same time, the nature of sleep cycles adds another level of complexity to sleeping together. If one of the couples is in the middle of a deep sleep cycle when awakened, they may find it difficult to adjust immediately and feel groggy and disoriented for several minutes. This disorientation could be the reason why you're getting out of bed on the wrong side!

When my alarm goes off in the morning, sometimes, it takes me forever to get my act together. I call it 'cotton wool brain', but it can sometimes last all

morning. A couple of times that I have been up early to take people to the airport, I have had to go back home and sleep more because I know I haven't actually woken up yet. I can drive and talk and do all that, but I'm not 100%.
Lulu, 42, legal professional, married 6 years

Similarly, being woken by a loud, unpleasant sound might just really annoy you, irrespective of in which sleep cycle you are.

My ex-boyfriend Brent wanted the radio alarm clock tuned to a hard rock radio station. I hated it. We agreed to swap every fortnight to the radio station of my choice, but on the mornings when a song I disliked (of which there were many) blasted me awake, it immediately put me in a bad mood. Similarly, the roles were reversed when my station was the wake-up call. Could we have chosen another way to wake up? Possibly, but two strong personalities don't always search for a rational solution. And my ongoing sleep deprivation from having to share a bed with him did not make me the most rational person at the time.
Wendy, 49, Communications

As mentioned in Chapter 2, sleep is regulated by two body systems—sleep/wake homeostasis and our circadian rhythm or body clock—and it is our circadian rhythm that dictates whether we are a morning person or evening person. 'Morningness' and 'eveningness' is in no small part, genetically determined. Therefore, if you are in a couple where there is a lark and an owl, your circadian rhythms are going to conflict. If one of you wants to go to bed and/or get up at the same time, there will have to be a negotiation of sleep timing and ultimately some form of compromise by one or both of you about when you go to bed and getting out of bed.

However, compromise just means there is the chance of one (or two) miserable people, e.g., if you're an owl going to bed too early, you are working against your circadian rhythm which means you are going to find it harder to fall asleep. Because your circadian rhythm is, to a large degree, genetically determined you cannot 'train' yourself to become a lark or an owl, although you can reduce the effects. For instance, owls would benefit from getting exposure to daylight as soon after they wake up as possible. Larks may find that getting out in the daylight late afternoon/early evening helps them to stay awake longer.

Meadows et al.[91] found that although couples went to bed at the same time, this was not necessarily their preferred bedtime "suggesting that couples do not necessarily want to go to their shared bed at the same time".

As with the 'in-bed' behaviours, there are more personal quirks and proclivities that manifest themselves in the bedroom and serve to disturb a sleeping, or attempting to sleep, partner. However, we will move on to the behaviours that some folk don't like to talk about in polite company, but we all know what happens when the sun goes down, and we head to our bedrooms.

The stuff we don't really like to talk about

There are some human bodily functions and activities that we all know about, but don't like to mention. A few of these activities take place in the bedroom, and the bed, and it's time to talk frankly about them.

Beeping your own horn

Animals do it. Humans do it. Apparently, humans do it on average 14 times a day. It's a natural bodily process of which we shouldn't be ashamed. It makes some people laugh uproariously and embarrasses others. It can be innocent and private or offensive and very public. Yep, we're talking about passing wind, or to be very blunt, farting.

On the list of bodily functions, we can't control, this one sits on the margins. While the passing of wind can happen unknowingly during sleep, we all know of people who boast of producing redolent emissions in the bed and the effect it has had on a poor, unsuspecting partner. But most of us have endured such behaviour and fail to see the humour. This does tend to be a behaviour that amuses and entertains men more than women – if you question my gender bias on this claim, just search 'farting in bed' on YouTube.

Unfortunately for men, physiologically they are more prone to farting because they generate more gaseous product in a day than women, and this gas is released when they are most relaxed. This, even more unfortunately for their partners, is likely to be in bed.

While farting when both parties are awake is terrible enough, farting while asleep constitutes cruel and unusual punishment.

Among a raft of behaviours that made me decide that I needed to sleep separately from my husband, his farting used to really, really irritate me. I should not have to put up with the smell of his fetid bowels when I am trying to go to sleep. As crude as that might be, it made me angry when he did fart in bed and even angrier when he thought it was funny. Even after six years of having separate bedrooms, he still thinks it amusing to come in to my bedroom at night, pass wind, and then leave me with the smell. There aren't words to capture how furious I become.
Holly, 33, British public servant

When sleeping with my husband, there is always the chance I will be woken by what I call a 'vivid' dream. I'm in a deep slumber and having an amazing dream and thinking 'Wow this dream is so real! I can even smell everything' only to be slowly drawn out of my slumber to find that the 'vivid' smell in my dream is, in fact, real and is coming from my perfectly undisturbed peacefully sleeping husband lying next to me! So after letting out a frustrating 'argh!' and purposefully waking up my husband giving him a good shove, because why should he have the luxury of sleeping while I have to deal with his smell, I grab my pillow in a fit of anger and traipse off to the spare room to try to salvage a few hours of solid sleep before my alarm is due to go off.
Emily, 30, international flight attendant, married 4 years

You know what? I sleep so much better when a man is not in my bed. My husband used to fart constantly, and it was really upsetting to me – smelly, gross and he stopped apologising too, so it was bad manners.
Anonymous, www.mamamia.com.au

I'd be happy with a separate room altogether. Who says love has to endure the cacophony of farts and snoring all night?
rhetoricalmuster, www.slate.com.au

It's one of life's little luxuries.
Ian, 42, electrician, married 5 years

Nothing says "I love you" like a 'dutch oven'
Lestroid, www.slate.com

The wet spot

When the activity and passion of sex are over, and a couple is basking in the afterglow of their encounter, there can be an issue that takes the shine off both love and lust – the wet spot.

For some couples, who sleeps in the wet spot is not an issue at all. The post-coital bliss may be so overpowering that falling asleep with each other comes naturally and without a second thought to the state of the sheets. But for others, it can make for an uncomfortable night's sleep – especially on cold winter nights.

The wet spot can vary in size, depending on the enthusiasm of the sexual act and if a condom was used.

So, if there is a moist area on the sheets, after each partner's breath has returned to normal and all the brain chemicals and feel-good after-effects of sex start to kick in, and sleep is washing over both of you, there is the inevitable battle of who gets to sleep in the dry part of the bed – or more importantly, who doesn't.

For those among us who are practical beings, preventative measures can be taken to mitigate the effects of the wet spot. Strategically placing a towel can help with absorption, but it's not very romantic and may take away from the spontaneity of the event. Having a spare sheet ready to pop on the bed quickly can also help, but again it's not really what most of us want to be doing after we've had sex.

Women may think that the chivalrous thing to do is for the man to offer up the dry area for his partner valiantly, but in these days of equality, that approach may be seen as untrue to the philosophies of the women's liberation movement.

Nine times out of ten, I will end up lying in the wet spot after sex. My partner falls asleep so quickly after sex, and it's a deep sleep that I can barely wake him from. I don't think he does it on purpose, but there have been many times that I have found a towel or a nightly to put over the spot, so it's not so 'icky'. I know it sounds a bit whingy, but after six years together the romance is waning a bit and it's hard to not get practical about these things.
Sam, 32, administrative assistant

My wife makes a bit of a deal about the wet spot

114

sometimes and will make me swap sides of the
bed so that I have to sleep in it. I fall asleep quickly
anyway, but I don't like not sleeping on my side of
the bed.
Ben, 36, builder

Sleeping separately will not completely stop the issue of the wet spot either – it just splits it across two beds. The problem that separately sleeping couples may face is whose bed is going to be subjected to the possibility of the wet spot.

There have been a couple of times after I have put
clean sheets on my bed that I have manoeuvred to
have sex with my husband in his bed rather than
mine. It took him a while to work it out, and then he
started doing it too. 'Whose bed will have the spot'
doesn't stop us having sex, but it makes choosing
the location a bit more strategic. We mostly laugh
about it.
Vicki, 46, executive officer, married 12 years

Baring it all

The last of the taboos to consider is what you wear to bed – or more specifically, what you don't. There's a spectrum of bed attire that runs from neck to ankle coverage, through to underwear such as pants and singlets and on to sleeping naked.

There are many reasons people give for sleeping naked:

- a level of freedom and comfort
- responding to and managing a high natural body temperature
- not having to deal with the hassles of nightclothes becoming tangled and uncomfortable
- the feeling of skin touching the skin of a partner
- less clothing to wash
- a general commitment to being naked.

If both parties are comfortable with the practice of sleeping nude, then all is well. But people who have been brought up with a certain level of modesty may find nudity in bed confronting and inappropriate. As with so many other aspects of our social being, we bring a sack full of moral and social beliefs to judge the behaviours of others. Any type of nudity can have a dramatic effect on those who were raised with the message that it is clothes on at all times of the day! Sometimes it's just that you don't like the feel of another person's skin in the same way that other people do.

> In 2002 I met my second wife, and we soon
> developed a very intimate relationship. She slept
> nude, all the time. It didn't matter if she had guests
> if the kids were around, or what, when she slid
> into bed, she slid in naked. I questioned her on
> this, and to my surprise, she thought I was the
> one that needed enlightening. She was right! I felt
> uncomfortable at first, sleeping nude with her both
> at her house and at mine. (I often slept over, and on
> occasion, she would sleep over with me.) But she
> didn't care; she wasn't going to wear anything and

be uncomfortable. So, I began to sleep nude, too.
Andy, 42, married for 6 years

*I stopped sleeping naked when I was with a boyfriend,
not because I didn't want to be naked, but because
he almost insisted that I sleep with clothes on. I don't
know what kind of message that is supposed to send,
but I'm not seeing him anymore, that's for sure.*
Libertine, 29, www.albertastars.com

*Being touched by my boyfriend's floppy penis at 2
am was never romantic or sexy. The reality, for me,
is that it affected my ability to be intimate. I found it
desensitising.*
Justine, 32, town planner

That is our tour through some of the realities of bed-sharing. We know the behaviours – both good and bad – discussed are not a complete list. This is because every couple is different and faces different challenges at different times in their life when it comes to why, how, and with whom they sleep. And it's the differences that are a critical factor in any discussion on the topic.

Each of the behaviours identified as 'bad' when it comes to sleeping with another person probably elicited responses that range from 'OMG – I totally get that, and it's the reason I can't sleep with my partner' through to 'OMG, I can't believe anyone could be that petty – get over yourselves and just go to sleep'. The purpose of naming these issues is to highlight that sleeping in a bed with another person night after night is not a simple task; that is, it is not a simple task for everyone.

As long ago as 2005 National Sleep Foundation Poll (America) revealed some interesting facts:[92]

- When one spouse has a sleep problem, 75% of their spouses end up with sleep problems too.
- If a spouse snores, the other spouse loses an average of 49 minutes of sleep each night.
- More than one-third of people with sleep issues say the issues caused problems in their relationship.
- One-quarter of spouses admitted that their sexual relationship had been affected by sleep issues.
- 23% of couples experiencing sleep problems end up in separate beds anyway.

Pause for thought…

- Do any of the behaviours outlined in this chapter keep you from sleeping at night? For example,
  - How many blankets/bedcoverings are on the bed?
  - How thick or thin is the quilt/duvet?
  - What temperature is the room?
  - Are the windows open or closed?
  - Is the fan on or off?
  - Is the air conditioning on or off? If it's on – what temperature?
- Have you spoken to your partner about what keeps you awake?
- How do you manage to get back to sleep if your partner disturbs your sleep?
- Are there nights where one of you has had to

find an alternative place to sleep because your partner's sleeping behaviours are keeping you awake? If so, do you have arrangements in place? What are they?
- Has either of your sleeping behaviours been the cause of arguments in your relationship?

FOUR

The Decision

'There is nothing in the world so difficult as that task of making up one's mind.'

Anthony Trollope[93]

In this chapter, we will discuss the issues around negotiating separate beds/bedrooms with your partner. However, one reason this may potentially be so difficult is the fact that, as discussed earlier, as couples, we rarely discuss our sleep with our partners. So, it might come as a bit of a shock to your partner that you are suddenly discussing—perhaps in some considerable detail—the causes and consequences of sleeping separately.

Until recently, there has been almost no research into the way couples negotiate their sleep together. However, in the last decade or so, sociological research has been conducted in this area with many of the, albeit limited numbers of, studies investigating couples sleep being performed by researchers from Sociology Department of the University of Surrey (Sara Arber, Jennifer Hislop, Rob Meadows, and Sue Venn) with whom Neil has been fortunate to collaborate and publish. Also, as mentioned earlier, social media platforms are being used more often to share separate sleeping arrangements, increasing to help the de-stigmatising of the practice.

When you start a relationship, you may discuss; where to live, how to share the bills, your hope and dreams and many other aspects of living together.

But as Jennifer Hislop[94] says "...couples rarely assess their compatibility as sleeping partners, choosing to share their nights with a partner despite the potential for disruption and poor sleep. Incompatibility in sleep behaviour and preferences may thus become a major source of tension over the life course of the couple relationship." Hislop also notes that "sleeping as a couple, while considered by some to be symbolic of a loving relationship, is fraught with the potential for sleep disruption". But our Western culture relationship aspirations don't seem to recognise or accommodate the fact that a couple can still be loving and not choose the potentially 'fraught' path of bed-sharing.

When you start a relationship, each partner brings to the relationship a view of both their sleep and the way to sleep with another person. This view is formed through the lens of their previous experience and expectations. We all have a life story, and the way we act and feel is developed based on our life's experiences. Thus, the expectations of our sleep needs are a product of numerous, often unknown, and unidentifiable, influences.

However, when we enter a new relationship, we now have another person's sleep to consider. Hislop[95] describes the situation thus, "......by being in a couple relationship, an individual's biological needs and right to a good night's sleep are potentially in conflict with both the needs of their partner and a commitment not to disturb their partner's sleep."

There are many aspects of the how, when, where of our sleep that need to be negotiated. Such aspects are:

- bedtime and wake up times
- bedtime routine
- which side of the bed to sleep on
- whether to have the windows open or closed or the heating on or off
- what type of mattress and pillows to have
- whether physical contact during the night is permissible
- the response to of snoring and other behaviours during the night
- and for parents – who gets up for the children during the night?

Reaching an agreement on these issues would be helpful to working out how a couple can get a good night's sleep that accommodates the needs of each partner. However, often these issues are not discussed and may become areas of conflict and resentment between the couple.

Further to this, rather than confront the problems, we may have a 'live and let live' or 'make do' attitude. In effect, we learn to put up with the other person's behaviour because we feel that sleeping together is more important than our individual need for sleep. Or as Hislop[107] puts it "couples are prepared to deprioritise their own sleep needs to ensure the maintenance of shared sleeping arrangements and as a symbol of the depth of their loyalty to the relationship."

Therefore, if we avoid negotiating our sleep role as a couple—which is the accepted norm for sleeping—it may be difficult to start discussing sleep with regards to sleeping separately after months, or years of sharing sleeping space. Where to sleep not only raises issues of intimacy, loyalty, etc., but also challenges custom, undermines expectations of social order, and risks moral censure.

In Chapter 3 we 'dived between the sheets' of the potential pitfalls of sleeping with another person, and highlighted that as couples, we might not be great at talking about our sleep needs or how our partner interferes with them. This may have you wondering then, where to from here? The answer to that question may, or may not, be quick and easy. As complex beings, we humans can surprise ourselves, and each other, with responses to unforeseen issues that arise when navigating the murky depths of relationships.

For some couples, the decision to amicably sleep apart is a no-brainer. It's sensible, practical, and logical, and poses no threat to the security of the relationship. For others, however, it raises deep fears that can manifest in feelings of rejection, guilt, betrayal, and shame. For some, the ritual and meaning of sharing a bed are so important that if this part of their relationship is challenged, the bedroom walls start collapsing around them.

Vive la différence!

Consider any advice from this book, or from other people you may discuss the topic with, within the context of your circumstances, your own needs, your partner's needs, and the needs of your relationship. These needs change, as you change, your partner changes, your life situation changes, your finances change, your career changes and … we're sure you get the picture. Everyone's relationship is bespoke – so make your decisions as unique as you are, and as tailor-made as haute couture.

This chapter summarises some of the key steps you can take to protect your relationship when making a difficult decision. We offer some tips along the way. These are intended to get you thinking about how you might begin to make the decision about changing your sleeping arrangements.

If you feel that raising the prospect of sleeping separately from your partner is going to cause a problem in your relationship, you need to be honest about this and decide why. For some couples, sleeping apart is a high-stakes decision – with potentially strong emotional responses to the suggestion.

To start, you might want to consider how much meaning is wrapped up in sleeping together (or apart) by you and your partner? For Jennifer and her husband, sleeping in the same bed every night wasn't all that important to either of them, so the meaning they attached to sleeping together was insignificant. However, the rules they created around spending time in a bed together and maintaining the rituals around goodnight and morning kisses were important because having a close physical relationship means a lot to them. For Neil, sleeping separately had come about because of not wanting to disturb his partner while working irregular hours as a sleep researcher. It was a pragmatic solution, but this meant that they had to be careful to ensure that intimacy was preserved. The emotion attached to the act of sleeping together each night will differ from one couple to the next. The vulnerability shown by sleeping next to another person is a sign of intimacy and great trust. So, if you no longer want to sleep with your partner, are you saying that you don't trust them and you don't want to share that level of intimacy anymore? When we can't separate the emotional from the practical, we run the risk of allowing fear of the unknown to develop into feelings of guilt and shame.

After knowing there are other people who sleep separately, I can finally let go of the guilt I felt about having separate rooms. I can barely function if I haven't had enough sleep and wake with a headache [that stays] for the whole day ... Some intimacy has been lost, but it's better than waking up angry every day.
Des, www.mamamia.com.au

We have only been sleeping in separate rooms for six months, but I still have a bit of guilt that this will eventually tear us apart. I rationalise this by thinking if we are going to be apart, we would be apart – this wouldn't be the thing that would cause it.
Anne, 44, senior manager, married 20 years

It was hard at first as I felt guilty. But once we got

into it and both felt so much better the next day after a good night's sleep, we just knew it was the right thing for us to do.
May, 66, retired, married 40 years

If sleeping separately is an issue because it negatively affects your relationship's security and stability, then it might be wise to look at that part of your relationship before deciding to sleep separately. It's a bit like buying a ticket for the Sydney Harbour Bridge Climb before finding out that you're afraid of heights. It is an excellent idea to do an inventory of the foundation of trust and commitment in the relationship before you climb up the hallway to the spare room.

While couples might have phases in their relationship where they take time out and sleep apart while resolving issues, sleeping apart permanently is a whole new ball game. Neither of us is a qualified relationship expert but are both confident that it is a good idea to have your relationship house in order before moving into the realm of separate bedrooms. Doing so will prevent the act of wanting to sleep separately from being confused with making a statement about other issues you might be dealing with together. So, before you start redecorating the spare room, you might want to consider what defines relationship success for you.

All the decisions we make in life are fundamentally driven by our priorities. Often these priorities are driven by our subconscious and don't reveal themselves explicitly, but they always influence our decisions. For example, if you are resolutely determined to lose weight, you are less likely to have a hamburger for lunch because your priority is to stop eating food that is high in calories. However, if you are feeling sad and find comfort in food, you may have a hamburger because your priority is to make yourself feel better through instant gratification.

After a previous failed relationship (nothing to do with sleeping) I knew that without sleep, I became a mess. The breakup was bitter and protracted, and the lack of sleep contributed to me developing a mild clinical depression. What I did learn though was that a big priority in my life was to always sleep well. That was non-negotiable. My new partner, who I love dearly, had a steep learning curve when coming to terms with that fact that I wasn't going to compromise on getting my sleep. We spend between three to five nights apart each week, and if I need it, sometimes, more. It was a tough reveal at the beginning of the relationship, but luckily he understands my situation. To be honest, he appreciates the fact that on the nights when he isn't sleeping all that well, he has the space and freedom to pop his laptop open and do some work or watch a movie to pass the time until he can fall asleep again.
Maddie, 35, health professional, married 6 years

We had been sleeping apart one or two nights a week throughout our whole relationship, but when the first baby came along, sleeping separately every night became essential. Each of us had reasons for absolutely having to get some sleep. As a surgeon, when I was operating the next day, I had to be well-rested. The other days, Maree needed to sleep so she could function well enough to look after the

baby and carry on with work. We simply took turns at sleeping in the room downstairs. It was very practical, and very necessary.
John, 33, married 3 years

Now that I've had the luxury of my own room and my own bed again, I won't be giving it up. I love shutting the bedroom door behind me and entering my own space to relax and ponder and rest. It sustains and nurtures me. There is nothing I like better than slipping into my bed each night, knowing I will sleep undisturbed until morning. Being able to spread out in a walk-in wardrobe is a definite plus as well. In time, if life does happen to bring a second partner for me, he will definitely need to be happy with a two bed/two room policy.
Veronica, 50, divorced after 25 years of marriage

If you plan to raise the topic of sleeping apart with your partner, this could be a good time to do an audit of what your priorities are in your relationship – and find out if they are the same as your partner's. Here is a simple exercise that provides some examples of relationship priorities.

Read the following statements then rate them, from YOUR perspective, in order of priority (1–10) according to how important YOU think they are to YOUR relationship. You can even consider just picking your top five priorities.

1. Our relationship is viewed as successful by others.
2. Letting your partner know that you love them every day is essential for a happy relationship.

3. Both people should always make important decisions in a relationship.
4. Spending quality time together every weekend is important.
5. Good, regular sex is an integral part of our relationship.
6. There should be an equal division of domestic duties between my partner and me.
7. Some form of close, physical contact with my partner every day is essential.
8. Agreeing on the financial aspects of our relationship is important.
9. A couple should never go to bed without resolving an argument.
10. A relationship should allow each person to have some space to do their own thing alone every week.

How do you think your partner would rate the statements? The same as you? Would you like to ask them to do the exercise? Then compare notes. Looking at the different ways you and your partner rate these activities might provide interesting insights for both of you.

– TIP 1 –
Take some time to work out the relationship priorities for you and your partner

---

The connection between relationship priorities and sleeping apart is very important. If your highest priority is to be able to sleep when and how you want so you feel rested and healthy, and your partner's priority is to sleep in the same bed because that equates to a successful marriage, then you will have a tough time reaching an agreement. Many people interviewed for this book hid their separate sleeping arrangements from family and friends because a priority for them was to present as a happy, normal couple. However, other couples were open about the practice because their priority was sleeping well and what other people thought about their arrangements was not important to them.

I have told one person at work that we have moved to separate rooms. I will never tell my parents. Why not? The social stigma that there's something wrong if you're not sleeping together. While I find the experience liberating, I don't think I will ever get comfortable about telling people.
Anne, 44, senior manager, married 20 years

I'm open about it because it just works fine for us. What I care most about is sleeping enough that I can deal with my life. I know we're okay.
Charlotte, 24, teacher, married 1 year

So, in your relationship, whose priorities are the right ones? Well, of course, neither and both. Each person's priorities are simply their priorities. If you start thinking in terms of right and wrong, it creates conflict or competition with your partner's priorities. However, these differences need to be discussed and clarified and sometimes compromise will be necessary. This doesn't necessarily mean someone has to give up their priorities – often a robust discussion and creative solutions can allow you to embrace both sets of priorities.

Another difference that affects people and can lead to conflict is having different needs. I might compromise on sleeping separately because your need for sleep is a high priority for you. However, you might compromise on telling friends we sleep separately because of my need to have this arrangement remain private. Needs also inform priorities.

Like many other topics touched on in this book, the issue of identifying, negotiating and managing priorities within your relationship can be researched through other means and is something you may want to look at, depending on your situation. Thinking about what your relationship and your priorities are, and how these sit alongside those of your partner, will help you to decide if separate rooms are going to be an option.

> *I moved to the spare room in our house as I could not sleep with my husband because of his snoring. He kept the main room, and I think I gave him the better room as I was the one leaving the shared bed. Why did I do this? Mainly the priority for me was getting sleep. Our new house will have two main rooms – both with ensuites, that's one of our new priorities.*
> Leanne, 41, HR executive, married 15 years

> *When I fell pregnant for the second time, I knew I needed to sleep every night. I am so tired; I am asleep by 7 o'clock every night. I need my sleep, and*

I need space so I can sleep diagonally across the bed; it's the only way I can get comfortable. He tries to sleep with me and complains there's no room, so I tell him to go to his own bed. He snores so loudly – like a tractor. I simply cannot function the next day if I sleep in the same bed as him. Maybe in the future, we might be able to sleep together, but at the moment, getting enough sleep is my priority, so it's separate beds.

Charlotte, 24, teacher, married 1 year

– TIP 2 –
Don't underestimate (or overestimate) the emotional response

If you haven't skipped directly to this chapter, you would have realised by now that you're not alone in having trouble sharing a bed and/or a bedroom. Even though a couple may be the consummate hosts at dinner parties, spend hours together happily tending their garden or make killer bridge partners, coming together in a small space every night, when both parties are at their most vulnerable because they are tired, may prove to be one of the tougher challenges you faced as a couple.

Issues around sleeping with another person can be just one person's, or they can be shared by both partners. Indeed, a shared problem will make the decision to sleep separately easier, but if you are fighting the battle alone, with a partner who wants to share a bed, then the path to separate slumber will be trickier to navigate.

My husband sees my inability to sleep in the same bed (because of his snoring) as my problem. He is happy to sleep with me, but I'm not [happy to sleep with him]. I feel that there has been a negative impact on the relationship, and it's seen as my fault. Over time he has come to understand how much we both value a good night's sleep though.

Amelia, 41, mother of two, married 12 years

I think he tried to take responsibility, but I don't think he fully understood how it was affecting me. The underlying feeling I had was he thought I was making it up.

Louise, 48, teacher, together 7 years

My husband is an insomniac, has been for years (since before we met), so there's not a simple solution regarding being stressed over something in particular. He would prefer to sleep alone, and there have been times when I've gone to the spare room, but I hate it. To me, that's housemates, not a marriage. I crave intimacy and feel rejected when he suggests I go to the spare room. He DOES love cuddling as much as me, before and after sleep, it's just the actual sleeping he'd rather do alone.

CJ, www.mamamia.com.au

Two years ago I told my partner I couldn't sleep in the same bed anymore. I was tired of the snoring, the fighting over the room temperature and the blankets. We now sleep in separate rooms, and I love it. Every once in a while she asks me to come back

and sleep with her, but I can't do it. We'll come into
each other's room for cuddling but leave each other
to sleep. It's saved our relationship. Sometimes the
romantic view of sleeping together gets lost in reality.
Chuck B, www.slate.com

How you approach a conversation about sleeping issues may differ depending on whether you are jointly or singly making the decision to sleep apart. However, what is similar in both scenarios is the initial honesty required to bring the problem out in the open.

How do you manage difficult conversations with your partner now? Is talking to each other about the tough stuff something you do easily, or does it take a crisis to bring feelings out into the open? Being honest with yourself about how you and your partner deal with high stakes decisions is a meaningful conversation you may need to have with yourself before settling down for a 'deep and meaningful'.

As has been noted, raising this topic is going to bring some emotions to the surface, no matter what the state of your relationship. Even when Jennifer and her husband were sleep-deprived and coming to the realisation they were going to have to sleep separately, making the first decision to just sleep apart during the week brought Jennifer to tears. She was scared about what this meant for their relationship as she had not thought for one minute that she would sleep separately from her partner. Were they strange? Could this work? Was it the beginning of the end after only six months? They were all valid questions at the time. In Neil's case, with his ex-wife and his current partner, sleep and the strength of his relationship were never really linked as sleeping separately was the default from the start of the relationships. You don't miss what you never had.

Years back, when we first made the decision to spend some nights apart, there was the question of 'Is this okay? Is it a harbinger of other problems?' But I think practicality won out at the end of the day.
Neil, 46, HR executive, married 19 years

When you have an emotionally charged discussion with your partner, do you always know how they will respond to a discussion of this nature? Can you confidently and safely predict the reaction when you give them bad news or news that is going to affect them adversely?

The longer you have been in a relationship, the more likely you will be able to predict your reaction and the reaction of your partner to these types of conversations. However, we often surprise ourselves at our reactions to specific events and news and cannot entirely predict the emotional response we will have. Afford your partner the same flexibility. Raising this topic may be more provocative than you think. So, while there is no way you can prepare for unexpected emotions and responses, being aware that the reaction might not be what you expect will at least allow you to be forewarned, if not forearmed.

– TIP 3 –
Plan how you will communicate with your partner about your issues around sleeping together

---

When you decide to raise the issue of changing your sleeping arrangements, may we start by cautioning against launching into the topic without some planning and preparation.

At an absolute minimum, it is not a good idea to open the conversation after you have spent another night thrashing around the bed due to your partner's snoring, teeth grinding or all-night movie watching. Chances are you won't be in the best frame of mind to raise the issue. Let's face it – you may not even have the power of adult speech. Being calm and coherent is a good foundation on which to begin a discussion. So at least wait until you are well-rested and in the realm of the rational.

Any marriage counsellor worth his/her qualification will tell you that solving problems in ANY relationship takes commitment, effort and a whole lot of patience, determination, and goodwill. So, when faced with the challenge of raising the issue of separate sleeping with your partner, go back to basics. The fundamentals for exploring the details of an issue are a good place to start getting your thoughts in order, so that's where we're going to start. The how, why, when, where, and what of talking to your partner about sleeping separately.

How?

As a starting point, you need to consider how you and your partner communicate. A good working relationship is based on effectively communicating all the time. But are you and your partner great communicators? And to be honest, how do you know for sure?

This book is certainly not going to delve into the theory of how couples should and do communicate. There are countless books, workshops, encounter weekends, and counsellors who can help you and your partner in that area. And to labour a point – because it's just so important – the way you and your partner communicate is going to be unique to you. One thing we do know from years of personal experience, is that sleeping separately requires vast amounts of communication.

I expect honesty and if my husband has a problem or issue, let's address it, talk about it and see what we can do. He has hinted that he wants us to sleep in the same room together to feel closer, but I like to sleep diagonally across the bed. We've talked about getting a king-sized bed, but then there's the issue of snoring, and I don't know how we're going to get around that – it's just too much. We do talk about it. We're open and honest about how we are feeling. I try to see things from his perspective, too. So it's just a matter of having open and honest communication. I can't read his mind, so he needs to feel confident telling me what he's thinking about our arrangements.
Charlotte, 24, teacher, married 1 year

When it comes to talking to your partner about changing a core tenet of your relationship, you need to be realistic. Don't set yourself up for disappointment. If having difficult conversations is not one of your strong points, then keep it simple. Don't assume you can have a profoundly intimate, nurturing dialogue if you've never had one before. Having a tough conversation successfully is a skill. That's why UN negotiators get paid a lot of money and consultants across the world make a fortune teaching other how to be great negotiators and have 'fierce' conversations. But they still get it wrong sometimes with their partners because of the unpredictability of a deeply emotional relationship.

Psychology 101 tells us that most people avoid awkward conversations with loved ones (and probably lots of other people) because it makes them feel uncomfortable. And as we pointed out earlier, sometimes we don't even know there's a difficult conversation we need to have. Unfortunately, if you avoid dealing with a troublesome situation, you may just be prolonging the agony and building resentment. Harbouring feelings of resentment against your partner is a danger to the health of your relationship. Feeling resentful of any person's behaviours can develop into slow-burning anger that doesn't do anyone in any relationship any favours.

I know that a contributing factor to the issues in our relationship is the fact that we don't talk to each other enough. We're not beyond fixing, but I get so angry that he won't talk about problems as readily as I do, and I know it's such a cliché because women want to talk more than men. He wasn't overly happy that we moved to separate rooms, but I've tried over and over again to explain to him how much better I feel now that I actually get some sleep at night. I feel guilty that he's not happy with our arrangement but am also a bit angry and resentful that he won't give anything to me that shows he understands my situation. I read a quote recently – 'Marriage is not a noun, it's a verb. It isn't something you get; it's something you do'. So, I guess we just keep on doing this marriage and work on the newer version of what was before. I just keep saying to myself 'back to the drawing board' to find a way to show him we can make this work.

Christine, 35, working mother, married 10 years

When sharing a confined space with another person, resentment can build for all sorts of reasons. A typical example is the friction that arises from differing approaches to routine domestic tasks. Who hasn't experienced, or caused, frustration with a partner for not taking out the garbage, not renewing the toilet roll, stacking or unstacking the dishwasher, not hanging towels up after use, leaving tissues in bed etc.

While these areas of potential conflict can be viewed as trivial, when silently fumed over and then bundled with other disparate, yet annoying behaviours and a bad day at work, we may find ourselves exploding in volcano-like proportions at the smallest of irritations, much to the bemusement of our partner, because the emotional pressure that has built up is akin to Mt Etna after a 50-year dormancy.

If your partner keeps you awake, or regularly disturbs your sleep, or interferes with how you want your bedroom's environment to be, and you don't tell them – how are they supposed to know?

I know I snore and am not proud of it. But I'm asleep, so how am I supposed to know what it's like to be

kept awake night after night? I'm asleep, but she thinks I should understand how she feels. I'm sorry, I just don't and yelling at me doesn't actually help.
Chris, 38, married 8 years

During menopause, my sleep became broken and increasingly elusive. While I could account for my mood swings, I thought my husband was having a phantom menopause because of his increasingly foul temper. After repeatedly questioning as to what was bothering him, he finally told me (yelled actually) that he hadn't slept properly for three months because of my newly developed erratic sleeping behaviour and furnace-like temperatures. Dumbstruck and just a little p***ed off, I pointed out that this was news to me and all he had to do was speak up. I felt embarrassed, furious, and helpless all at the same time. I wish he had told me in a kinder way, realising that it was uncontrollable by me and equally as annoying. He said he didn't know how to bring the subject up as he too was embarrassed. Honestly, 29 years of marriage and you would think we could get this stuff right between us.
Nicola, 55, retail manager, married 29 years

If not sleeping at night is affecting you negatively and you feel it's a problem, then, simply, it is a problem.

Some couples speak proudly of their excellent 'bed life' and how they just soldier on with each other's little quirks in bed because that's what good couples do. These conversations can make you think that you should try harder and learn to cope with broken sleep because other people seem to be able to do it. However, if disrupted sleep prevents you from functioning at work, and with life in general, know that it is enough of an issue to raise in your relationship.

The challenge can be trusting your feelings, clarifying these feelings for yourself, finding the words to clearly explain your situation and then working out how to articulate this to your partner in a loving way that makes them believe you. This is easy to say, but not so easy to do.

> *My husband was unhappy that I was sleeping on the couch every night. He told me he felt that we were flatmates with benefits. But his snoring and restlessness was keeping me awake every night and I couldn't function well enough to look after our children. I just sat him down to have a talk about it and showed him some bruises from where he had 'hit' me during the night and he was devastated. I knew we needed to have a purposeful conversation about the situation, and I don't think you can work through an issue like this unless you have that conversation. After the talk, he understood why I had made the decision, but the honest talk is needed.*
> Caroline, 30, photographer, married 7 years

We all like to feel valued and acknowledged by significant people in our life – especially our partner. Frustration can build when we tell another person how we feel, and they don't believe us. Having concerns dismissed by another erodes trust and respect in a partnership.

If your partner does not believe that your sleep is

being disrupted, you may need to find ways of clearly and calmly proving your reality. Simple tactics such as having a third party confirm your assessment of the annoying behaviour, recording a snorer, taking photographs of extreme sleeping positions, or keeping a journal of when your partner wakes you can help. If you are desperate, you could perhaps employ the devices used in the Paranormal movies and set up a camera. While these tactics might seem extreme, hard facts make for more productive conversations than relying on anecdotes and emotionally charged tales of woe.

> *We recently shared a hotel room with a good friend to save on costs, and when said friend fell asleep and promptly began snoring, my husband was amazed that anyone could put up with it. And he thought I'd been exaggerating all these years – it was good for him to get his own medicine!*
> Sash, www.mamamia.com.au

> *It might sound childish, but I recorded my husband's snoring on my phone when he continued to suggest that I was exaggerating the volume and ferocity. I titled it 'The Lion Sleeps Tonight' and felt a degree of satisfaction when he was stunned into silence when watching it. Our conversations about how I couldn't get much sleep certainly changed after that.*
> Lulu, 42, legal professional, married 6 years

> *I decided my boyfriend needed to see the carnage caused at night from his bed acrobatics so every time I woke because the covers had been wrenched*

from me again, or he'd done another tumble turn and rolled on to my side of the bed, I got up, turned on the light and woke him to point out the state of him and the bed. The first night he thought it was a bit entertaining because he would just go back to sleep, but by about the fourth night, he started to get cranky with me. But it wasn't over. By night six, he agreed that being woken multiple times every night was not much fun.

Justine, 32, town planner

While honesty – both in facts and feelings – is an important part of why you are raising this subject with your partner, don't use it as an excuse for disrespect and contempt, or as a chance to take a swipe at your partner for something else, under the guise of separate sleeping. It's true that you need to express how you feel to your partner and tell them the truth, but you also need to consider the other person's feeling when choosing your words as once you've said something – there's no taking it back. And maybe avoid the excessive use of adjectives when describing the behaviour.

Douglas Stone, Bruce Patton and Sheila Heen's book, *Difficult Conversations: How To Discuss What Matters Most*,[96] provides insights into why people fail to communicate on difficult topics. Their book identifies three sub-conversations that take part in any difficult conversation. One of these sub-conversations – 'The "What Happened?" conversation – considers where the truth lies in a contentious issue and how agreed facts might mean something completely different to each party.

You will have your truth about what is happening in

bed every night – as will your partner. You will also have your version of what needs to happen to address the issues you have in bed every night – as will your partner. I am sure you have had discussions with your partner where your versions of events do not match, but you are both vigorous in defence of your version as the most truthful and accurate account. Sound familiar?

Truth is an interesting concept. We all feel confident our version of life is THE truth. Unsurprisingly, our view of the world can tend to be a tad self-centred as human beings are driven by ego and a basic instinct to fight for what we believe is right. The lens that we view life through is shaped by values, morals, judgements, cultural twists, and social mores. We also tend to believe that we know why other people are making choices that affect us because we try and rationalise their behaviour by thinking about what we would do in that situation. This thinking on behalf of others is a recipe for disaster.

Both common human behaviours can lead us on a trip down Disaster Road if we construct the contents and the outcomes of a discussion without genuinely considering the other person's input. Patton and Heen give three pointers when dealing with the 'facts' of a difficult conversation.

- **The Truth Assumption** – we often fail to question one key assumption – 'I am right, you are wrong'. There's only one hitch: I am not always right. Difficult conversations are almost never about getting the facts right. They are about conflicting perceptions, interpretations, and values. They are not about what is true, but about what is important.

- **The Intention Invention** – the error we make is simple: we assume we know the intention of others when we don't. Intentions are invisible, so we make them up based on what we know.
- **The Blame Frame** – the third error we make is that most difficult conversations focus significant attention on who's to blame for the mess we're in. Talking about blame distracts us from exploring why things went wrong and how we might correct them going forward. Focusing on the conversation instead allows us to learn about the real causes of the problem and to work on a plan to correct them.

Before deciding that you know what's going wrong and then possibly how you can fix it, try to develop a curiosity about your partner's version of events, so you are confident your ideas won't create an even bigger problem because you have the facts wrong. Do you even know if sleeping together is an issue for them or if it's a topic they are prepared to discuss?

Simple questions that are an excellent way to start a conversation include: 'How well do you think we sleep together?' or 'If you had one concern about our sleeping behaviours/ patterns, what would it be?' or 'What would you say if I told you that I'm not getting enough sleep each night?'

How your partner communicates is yet another consideration you need to throw into the mix. Keep their style in mind. People feel less threatened if you can communicate in a way that is familiar and comfortable to them. If your partner likes facts, give them facts. If they want detail, tell the story. If they respond to an emotional take on the topic, then wear your heart on your sleeve. Some people just want to get straight to the solution and what it means for them, so make sure you get through to at least the end of this chapter so you can begin to articulate what it is that you want.

Thomas Bradbury and Benjamin Karney, authors of *Intimate Relationships*,[97] make the point that in a relationship, disagreement is inevitable, but conflict is optional. This is based on a theory where strong, clear communication takes the place of blame laying, finger-pointing and aggressive, thoughtless fighting. There might be times when talking about separate sleeping that you don't agree with each other or feel emotional about the topic, but avoiding a situation where you conflict is undoubtedly preferable. Again, if you need more information about communicating with your partner, further reading or support from a counsellor or psychologist might be worthwhile.

– TIP 4 –
Clearly, factually, and calmly explain why your partner's behaviour is disturbing your sleep.

Why?

While this might seem like an obvious question, does your partner really understand why their behaviour is disturbing your sleep? They might know that you are cranky with them in the morning because they snore, or accidentally end up with the covers on their side of the bed, but have you calmly and with sufficient detail explained the effect of their behaviour on you? What is it about their bed behaviours that interfere with your sleep at night?

It's recommended that you take some time to think about how you might be able to clearly articulate why you find sleeping with your partner difficult. Think about how you could explain how their behaviour affects YOU, rather than making accusations that blame them for their behaviour. The examples in the table on the next two pages might help. Remember that many annoying, nocturnal behaviours are not a choice people make. They are just part of the wonderful array of characteristics that make us all unique and are mostly unintentional.

When we know how our behaviour is affecting others, we are more inclined to change it, depending, of course, on how much we care about the other person.

If you have a partner, who is inclined to be a bit less considerate or flexible, convincing them that their behaviour is impacting negatively on you and then having them care enough to change could be your particular challenge.

Sharing a bed just wasn't working. He would get up between 4–5 am every morning, and then he would go into the ensuite bathroom and put the light on. So all the things that I didn't do to let him sleep when I came to bed later than him each night, he was just marching on and doing regardless of the fact it woke me up. Therefore, resentment was building up with me, and because he was the one that went to bed early, he was always in control. I would feel guilty and uncomfortable going into the room, turning a light on

and sitting up reading if he was asleep – but that type
of behaviour didn't seem to bother him.
Kaye, 66, together 14 years

Unfortunately, there is no quick or easy answer for dealing with a self-centred partner. There are many reasons why some people are less inclined to be considerate than others. Our guess is that if your partner is not considering your needs in the bedroom, they are likely to be this way in other areas of your shared life.

The table opposite shows some examples of how you can reframe statements about how your partner's behaviour is affecting your sleep.

Can you see the difference? One statement has the potential to make your partner feel bad and has a strong possibility of putting them on the defensive because they feel under attack. The other might help them understand the issue from your perspective. Merely naming the behaviour, without explaining the problem from your perspective and the impact it has on you does nothing to increase your partner's understanding of your situation.

Communicating with your partner is the way to address this concern and is well outside the scope of our advice – but we do wish you well in helping them to understand that you too have rights when it comes to sleeping each night.

– TIP 5 –

Plan when and where you will have the conversation so that your partner will be at his or her most receptive.

What you might feel like saying to your partner	What you might choose to say instead
Honey, your snoring is driving me insane! I can't get any sleep!	I'm such a light sleeper that your snoring keeps waking me during the night, and I'm not getting enough quality sleep to function properly.
Why should I have to wear earplugs every night so you can lie there and snore like a rhino?	Even though I can sleep through your snoring when I wear earplugs, I can do it for a while, but after about three days they irritate my ears, and then I can't sleep because of the irritation.
If you steal the covers off me one more time, I swear I'm going to kill you	When you toss and turn in bed, you often move the covers so much that I don't have any, and then I get cold and wake up. Because it happens a few times each night, my sleep is broken, and this makes it hard for me to keep up with the kids the next day. It makes me grumpy and resentful. I don't want to feel like that, but it's what happens when I can't sleep.
Stop getting up SO many times during the night; it's really, really annoying. Why can't you just go to bed and stay in bed? I can.	When you get up during the night, you disturb my sleep. I find it hard to fall back to sleep because I lie awake, thinking about when you will get out of bed again.
How about you just marry your laptop/smartphone, so you never have to be apart?	When you use your laptop in bed at night, the movement from you typing and the noise, even though it's not really loud, keeps me awake. I really need to get a good 7–8 hours of sleep every night so that I can think clearly at work
WOULD YOU JUST STOP FARTING WHEN YOU ARE ASLEEP!!! DO YOU HAVE DEAD ANIMALS IN YOUR BODY?	Were you aware that the smell from your farts is so strong that it wakes me up? I get really upset, and I find it hard to get back to sleep because I am so angry that I'm awake and you're still asleep.

When and where?

We've put 'when' and 'where' together as they are common bed partners in this problem-solving framework. The location of your chat may be heavily influenced by the time it takes place and vice versa – you may choose a particular time to have a conversation, and this may dictate where it happens. As touched on earlier, your best bet is to raise the issue at a time when both of you are in a rational frame of mind and in a location that is conducive to a productive, adult conversation.

When I screamed at my husband at 2.30 am one Friday morning that I couldn't sleep with him anymore, I don't think it really had the best outcome – initially. I was having a crappy week at work, stressed trying to have a report finished for Friday afternoon, Greg [my husband] was snoring worse than normal with a cold, when he wasn't snoring, he was coughing, and I just lost it. All he could talk about though was how sick he was feeling and how thoughtless I was. This made the situation worse for me, and I ordered him out of the bed. We didn't talk much over the weekend and, yes, I know it wasn't the best way to raise the topic of sleeping apart. But hey, I'm human.
Maria, 38, database analyst, married 8 years

I had a really bad cold, was having trouble sleeping and Maria thought it was a good idea to wake me at some ridiculous time, shrieking at me for snoring or something. I told her she was thoughtless as it was me who was sick, and I needed my sleep to

get better. I get that I have to talk about stuff in our
marriage, but I did suggest she could pick her times
a bit better. I do remember being particularly p***ed
off with her for a few days.
Greg, 39, engineer, married 8 years

Realistically, the issue of disturbed sleep is unlikely to be solved with one conversation. Consciously choosing when and where you will raise the topic is a wise move. As Greg and Maria illustrate, raising the topic when either of you is tired and not thinking rationally is not a recommended approach for success.

When buying a house, your focus is location, location, location. When raising a tricky topic with your partner, focus on timing, timing, timing – and location. Be sensible and use some logic about when you bring up the topic. For example, don't try and strike up a conversation with them when they are on their way to or from work, they have just sat down to watch their favourite show on television, or they have scheduled something that you know about, and the talk will keep them from getting there on time.

You know the times when your partner is at their best and worst, so maximise your chance of success and pick a time they are likely to be at their best.

Depending on their temperament, you may even choose to warn your partner that you want to have a chat about something. It may prevent them from feeling ambushed, or because they were not aware you wanted to talk, arrange to be out somewhere or doing something else.

And as for the where, think carefully. If you are thinking

of using a public place, for example, a restaurant or a public walkway, do consider your partner's needs. If their emotional response is strong, being in a public place may make them feel defenceless and detract from the chance of getting a positive outcome from the conversation.

Lying in bed on a Saturday or Sunday morning could be precisely the time you know your partner is at their most rested and communicative. For some couples, a post-coital chat could provide the necessary intimacy to raise an issue such as this as there is often a deep feeling of trust after a couple has had sex.

We could give more examples of when and where might be good, but the reality is that you know the answer to these two pieces of the puzzle better than anyone. If you are reading this and thinking 'there is never a good time', then we suggest you bite the bullet, take your chances, and pick what you believe to be possibly the time and place for you to manage the conversation to the best of your abilities and talents.

– TIP 6 –
Be honest when considering the positives and negatives of changing your sleeping arrangements.

What?

Of all the questions to prepare for, we think this is the most important: 'What do you want?'

Do you even know what you want? Are your thoughts limited to 'I just need to get some sleep every night' or have you spent a lot of time thinking about how you might re-engineer your current sleeping arrangements to make everyone's life better?

As the person raising the issue, you do have a responsibility to take the lead on how the 'new world' is going to look. Simply saying 'I can't sleep with you' is probably going to limit the scope of your partner's response options and may also limit your opportunity to manoeuvre the conversation towards the outstanding plan you have devised to solve your sleeping troubles.

In planning to raise this issue with your partner, be very clear about what you are trying to achieve. Do you just want to open the discussion on the problems you have when you sleep with your partner? Or are you seeking to find and put in place a solution that involves changing the current sleeping arrangements? Be honest, do you just want the problem as you see it acknowledged, or are you well past that and pining for your own space every night?

Even though you might think you have all the answers and the 'best solution ever', you need to be prepared to concede that this may not be the way your partner sees it – in fact they may think it is the 'worst solution ever' – especially if they have not been involved in any of the thinking and planning for the change.

This may surprise you, but what you see as the solution to your problem is probably going to have positive and negative consequences. Just the same as staying in a bed with a person who keeps you awake all night has negative consequences, moving into another room might have some negatives too. As a rational and reasonable person, be prepared to admit to the negatives – ignoring them is foolhardy. We all know that not every decision ends in a win-win situation. It's tough, but that's life. Make sure you are clear and honest about all aspects of the decision, all plusses and minuses, as it will make for a more balanced and complete discussion.

– TIP 7 –

Be able to describe to your partner exactly what the change to your sleeping arrangements is going to look like, what the change to your relationship is going to look like and be open to their suggestions too.

Don't limit yourself to thinking there is only one answer to your problem/s. Depending on how your partner is disturbing you, there might be a range of options that you can suggest or that your partner might offer in reply, once you open the dialogue. And if your ultimate goal is for separate rooms, you may need to consider some interim steps along the way.

We were both exhausted, cranky, sleep-deprived parents of two energetic boys struggling to keep up with life. We discussed sleeping in separate beds for a few days a week to catch up on sleep, and a few days turned into weekdays, then we would try to sleep together on weekends, but that still didn't work so we have very happily been getting a lot more sleep and having a happier, healthier and better relationship in the years since we decided to separate – our beds, that is. We both highly

Admittedly, for some bed-sharing incompatibilities, sleeping in a separate room might be the only option available, but get creative and be open to a range of suggestions.

Chapter seven explores the range of options as alternatives to hopping into the same bed every night, but finding the right option for you might come down to deft negotiation skills.

Your particular circumstances may require one or a combination of solutions. For example, sleeping in separate rooms three to four nights a week, and then no television on the nights you sleep together. But whatever solution you do come to, it's important to remember:

- don't focus on only one option as it may not be the only one (or the right one)
- get creative and investigate several options that may be available
- be prepared to try a few options – especially if your partner has suggested some.

You may even consider talking to other people about your situation as they may see a solution that you can't.

The next part of winning your partner over to the new world order is considering how the changed arrangements will affect your relationship. If your partner has a strong attachment to the practice of sleeping together every night, be prepared to describe what your relationship is going to look like – and not just the physical sleeping arrangements.

Tina B Tessina, an American psychotherapist points out that, 'Couples who choose sleeping apart need to make an extra effort to connect every day and be physically close in whatever way possible. It's already difficult for most couples to find time to discuss things, keep up to date with each other and solve problems together – three main functions of a working marriage – sleeping apart adds one more obstacle to the mix.'[98]

If your partner foresees a loss of intimacy and physical contact as a result of sleeping apart, and then equates these perceived losses the start of the end of the relationship, you need to find ways to reassure them that is not the outcome you foresee or want. What will you be able to tell your partner about the new version of your relationship that will reduce concern? Remember, just because you have something in mind, doesn't mean that your partner shouldn't have input.

Have you thought about how the loss of physical contact is going to be addressed if you move in to separate rooms?

If you think that you don't care about this – all you want is a good night's sleep – you may find that when you are well-rested and feeling a little more in control that you do want to connect with your partner physically. This is why keeping all options and possibilities about your physical relationship uppermost in discussions is a crucial part of managing this change. As many couples' report that a good night's sleep rekindles their relationship, you may want to ensure that whatever you negotiate in terms of new sleeping arrangements doesn't shut the door to maintaining or improving the physical part of your relationship.

So, what does your future look like in terms of sleeping arrangements? And if they are going to change dramatically, how can the physical and emotionally intimate parts of the relationship be cared for? That is up to you.

Every couple has different ways of staying connected based on what is important to them as individuals, as a couple and as a family. What you do in terms of managing your sleeping arrangements and managing your relationship to cater for those changes requires thought, planning, sensitivity, creativity, and a commitment to the cause.

– TIP 8 –

Get ready for the sex talk – be able to explain how you think sleeping separately might affect your sex life (don't forget to accentuate the potential positives).

One of the trickiest problems to tackle when raising the prospect of sleeping apart is dealing with the question of 'What is going to happen to our sex life?' This aspect is, but not exclusively, a more significant concern for men.

Later in this chapter, we discuss the fact that we are the only species that equates sex with being in bed and then falling asleep. And herein lies another social construct – the one that associates a successful sexual relationship with sharing a bed every night. Klösch[99] describes the association of 'sleeping together' with 'being sexually active', and there is undoubtedly a cultural implication that if a male and female share a bed, then there is the chance of sexual activity. Neil has made the point that 'sex and sleep are entirely separate entities, whereas we have put them into almost the same activity where if you are not sleeping next to somebody, then you are not having sex with them, and that is just foolish in the extreme. It doesn't make sense.'[100]

Because of the cultural connotations, we place on 'sleeping' with another person there is often an underlying suggestion that you might 'get' or be expected to engage in sex when you hop into bed with each other. The expectation that 'bed = sex' puts another layer of complexity in place for those who look to their bed as a place of rest after a busy day. Stephanie Coontz suggests the idea that a person should be permanently turned on and permanently available is an unnecessary burden for modern couples. She also challenges the assumption that if you choose to sleep in another room, away from your partner, you're maybe not very sexual.[101]

My sons have all said to me that if I'm not there when dad wants sex, there'll be problems. Good luck to him, I say.
Von, 72, married 55 years

I think the issues around why people are concerned that you're not sleeping in the same bed are more about sex. If you are not sleeping with each other, then other people assume you are not having sex. People feel the need (men particularly) to say they

are having a lot of sex. We have a saying – 'We have
full visiting rights, but then he can f*** off when he's
done.'
Melissa, 47, executive, married 27 years

Most likely, you and your partner started your relationship with passionate, lustful sex where you couldn't wait for the opportunity to be in bed together. But science and sociology tell us that these lustful ways naturally wane as a relationship progresses, children come along, responsibility kicks in, and we find a sexual routine that fits in around the busyness and complexities of our lives.

Do you think that sleeping separately will affect your sex life? Are you able to articulate your thoughts about any possible effects of sleeping separately on your sex life? Can you share these with your partner? Remember, the consequences might be positive.

Some couples don't feel comfortable talking about sex and think that sex should just happen naturally – no communication required to ensure that each partner is happy, satisfied and having their needs met. If this sounds like you and your partner, then moving to separate rooms to sleep may create uncertainty for you both about how sex will still happen.

So, whether you plan to suggest that you would like to move out of the bedroom permanently, or just sometimes, you may want to include your sex life on the discussion agenda. Even a gentle quip about having visiting rights or 'your bed or mine' could help to put a nervous partner's mind at ease and reassure them that you can't foresee any drastic changes to the current 'sextus quo'.

On a practical level, you are probably heading into

uncharted territory with this suggestion, so the truth is that you may not even know what your sex life will be like if you move to another room. (There are some suggestions in Chapter 6 if you want to skip ahead and get some pointers for your chat.)

Sleeping separately certainly does not mean an end to, or even an interruption to, your sex life. In fact, many couples report an improved sex life after moving to separate rooms, mainly because having a sufficient sleep every night means they aren't so grumpy and tired, and as a result, they feel like sex more often. (They also feel more loving and receptive because they no longer want to physically harm their partners because of night after night of pent-up resentment and anger.)

This fact may be a good starting point for a discussion about why moving to separate rooms might even improve your sex life.

Many women report that having their own space means that they don't feel like they are 'on tap' all the time for sex with their partners. In discussing this issue in her book, A Strange Stirring, Stephanie Coontz[102] reported that several women spoke of the pressure to always be in the same bed was bad for their sex life because it made sex sort of routine, instead of making the choice and an effort to initiate it. The outcome of sleeping separately maybe that sex becomes more exciting because it's not just a matter of 'Oh, you're there, so let's do it' but more sought after and deliberate.

*My husband and I have an intentional intimacy now.
Moving to separate rooms after being together for 24
years has actually made our sex life more exciting –*

it's removed the obligation of just going to bed and finding each other. Now we visit the other's room, and it feels more special.
Anne, 44, senior manager, married 20 years

We sleep better in separate beds and we both know it, but we are nonetheless enslaved by this stupid idea that if we don't share the 'marital bed' we are somehow dysfunctional. As if the bed is the only place to have sex. As if we only have sex at night, with the lights off. It's hooey.
Peregrinus, www.slate.com

If you tie your sex and intimacy to being in bed at night together, sure, you will have less. My husband and I are more rested and happier sleeping in different rooms. That has led to a far more robust and intimate life as a whole.
nooneparticular, www.slate.com

Because we both get a good night's sleep, we argue less because we have the patience to work through our problems better than we used to. Because of this, we seem to have become more tactile with each other, and simply, this has led to more sex. We're not doing it all the time, but I would definitely say we have more sex than we were having, say, about four years ago.
Mike, 52, landscape gardener, married 23 years

Bed's not the only place to have sex. I would feel like I'm from the 1950s if I went to bed every night

and just expected that sex was going to happen.
Sleeping separately certainly stops the '2 ams' and I
no longer have to deal with the 'tap on the shoulder'.
But we have a very active sex life. I'm happy, and I
know he's happy.
Amelia, 41, mother of two, married 12 years

There is an increasing number of couples embracing the concept of date nights, and there is no reason why this can't continue through to arranging a romantic tryst with your partner where you invite them to your room on Friday or Saturday night for a 'date night with benefits'.

Realistically, when it comes to sex – depending on the level of importance placed on it by you and your partner – sleeping separately could prove to be just what you are looking for to give your sex life a shot in the arm, rather than it sounding the death knell to this part for your relationship.

This statement is not a joke; we provided some statistics about the impact of sleep deprivation on how couples function in Chapter 2. Research shows that poor sleep interferes with our ability to manage conflict in relationships and essentially makes us more likely to fight with our partners. Researchers at the University of California, Berkeley[103] investigated the association between poor sleep and conflict in romantic relationships and their study revealed that couples reported more conflicts in their relationships on days that followed poor nights of sleep. Just a single night of poor sleep was associated with increased relationship conflict, even for those people who were generally good sleepers.

They also found that poor sleep was associated with

more negative feelings between partners. Even when one partner reported sleeping poorly, both partners were more likely to report and display greater negative feelings. Couples also exhibited less empathy towards each other and were less skilled at reading each other's emotions when one or both partners slept poorly. And poor sleep made conflict resolution more difficult.

In a separate study, researchers at the University of Pittsburgh School of Medicine[104] found that better sleep at night predicted less negativity between partners the following day. They also found that positive daily interaction between partners predicted better sleep quality at night. And finally, on this point, researchers from the University of Nebraska-Lincoln and Brigham Young University[105] found that couples with different sleep-wake routines, e.g., an early riser married to a night owl, experienced more conflict, spent less time in shared activities and conversation, and had sex less often than couples whose sleep-wake habits were aligned.

So, anything that improves your sleep — including sleeping apart — will enhance your ability to function as a couple successfully and harmoniously and make it easier for you to negotiate with each other. It is not for nothing that this book is called 'Sleeping Apart not Falling Apart'.

We hope the last couple of chapters have provided you with some background information about sleeping behaviour and a simple framework to organise your thoughts and plan a strategy to have a discussion with your partner about your sleeping issues. Having tough conversations with anyone isn't easy. Humans like to protect those close to us, and that protection extends to emotional safety. If you can find the right words to say at the right time, you may find that potential hurt is minimised, and you can achieve a much-needed level of honesty.

Now let's see what the outcome of your discussions might look like as a negotiated agreement.

Tip Summary

Tip 1   Take some time to work out the relationship priorities for both you and your partner.

Tip 2   Don't underestimate (or overestimate) the emotional response.

Tip 3   Think about and plan for how you will communicate with your partner about your issues.

Tip 4   Clearly, factually, and calmly explain why your partner's behaviour is disturbing your sleep.

Tip 5   Plan when and where you will have the conversation so that your partner will be at their most receptive.

Tip 6   Be honest when considering the positives and negatives of changing your sleeping arrangements.

Tip 7   Be able to describe to your partner exactly what the change to your sleeping arrangements is going to look like, what the change to your relationship is going to look like and be open to his suggestions too.

Tip 8   Get ready for the sex talk – be able to explain how you think sleeping separately might affect your sex life (don't forget to accentuate the potential positives).

Pause for thought...

- How well do you and your partner communicate with each other?
- Do you ever discuss how (not if) you communicate?
- Have you and your partner talked about what your sleeping issues are and how they could be resolved?
- How do you and your partner communicate about your sex life?
- What happens in your 'home' when one person wants something the other doesn't? How do you let each know what you want?
- If you know you aren't great communicators and have unresolved problems in your relationship, have you ever considered seeking external help to assist you in communicating better?

FIVE

Negotiating the outcome

'Everything is negotiable. Whether or not the negotiation is easy is another thing.'

Carrie Fisher[106]

Once you feel you have covered the how, why, when, where, and what of bed-sharing, then you need to prepare for the outcome of your discussions. Are you and your partner able to negotiate a mutually acceptable decision about changed sleeping arrangements with which you can both live? Take a deep breath and begin.

If you both agree that your sleeping arrangements need to change, consider yourself fortunate. And if you can immediately concur on how the new arrangements will work, then bravo! The ability of couples to find solutions to tough problems is dependent on a vast array of variables and managing those variables will no doubt remain a great source of income for psychologists and self-help authors for years to come.

As noted, it's tough to hear someone else's view of, or solution to, a problem when you know you have the answer. It's even tougher when the other person doesn't see how fantastic your solution is and has the audacity to challenge, pull apart or even refuse to agree with your insightful and well-crafted plan. When they do come up with an alternative or fail to agree to your brilliance, what are you going to do?

As mentioned earlier, a component of problem-solving for couples is having and then exhibiting goodwill. But what exactly does that mean? Words and phrases used to explain goodwill include benevolence, kindness, friendliness, cheerful acquiescence, consent and a favourably disposed attitude towards. They all mean the one thing – playing nice while agreeing to something you may not necessarily want to agree to. Ow! Negotiation hurts!

Having goodwill is a state of mind. It's a willingness to enter into something with your best manners, your best attitude, your nicest words, and a healthy dose of care and concern for the other person with whom you are negotiating. This care and concern need to centre on finding an outcome that works for them as well as you so that it really is the best outcome.

I think my husband understood I could no longer physically sleep next to him. He has mentioned a few times that he misses me. He sleeps better when I am next to him; he can go back to sleep better when

I am next to him. When he asked if we could ever sleep together again, I said, 'If you can do something about your snoring, then maybe we can' – but I would not expect him to go through the operations needed to fix the snoring. Three of them didn't work for my mother. How did I feel when he said that? Nostalgic, because I knew it would never happen. Quite honestly, I can't sleep next to a log cabin being built with logs being sawn all night.

Suzette, 40, administrative assistant, married 17 years

There is much that has been researched and written about the outcomes and purpose of negotiation. Business and diplomatic negotiations have serious terms such as 'distributive', 'integrative', 'interdependence', 'leverage' and 'strategic'. While negotiating with your partner need not involve the high-level theoretical knowledge and skills of a UN diplomat, there are aspects of formal negotiation that are worth considering.

Two notions are particularly useful: 'Negotiation is the principal way that people redefine an old relationship that is not working to their satisfaction' and 'The goal of negotiation is not to win, it is to succeed'. Both are precisely what you are aiming for – a successfully redefined relationship.

Our fundamental survival instinct as humans, keeps us bound to our self-interest, and appropriately so. This practice served us well in our early days of fending off wild animals and foraging for food in the pursuit of basic survival. So, it's natural that we continue to manoeuvre and arrange our lives to meet our own needs. But when we must accommodate other people who don't have precisely the same plans that we do, then we must find ways of manoeuvring to keep as much of our planned outcome as we can.

To help you negotiate with your partner to change your sleeping arrangements, we offer three potential strategies. We're going to offer them in the order of least favourable to most likely to succeed. They are sacrifice, compromise, and consensus.

Sacrifice

In this book, we use sacrifice in the context of when one person gives up something important or valuable so that another person can have something else. (Just wanted to clarify that in case anyone thought we might be suggesting the ritual killing of another human – in this case for the crime of keeping you awake for five nights in a row by snoring loudly – a fundamental distinction.)

All close and long-term relationships require a degree of sacrifice. It's a behaviour that oils the wheels of marriages, friendships, work relationships and parenting. In fact, many people might see sacrifice as the ultimate expression of love for another person and sometimes it is. When we give up something we want, e.g., to eat Thai takeaway instead of pizza, we do so because we are invested in a relationship and understand that part of socialising successfully in that relationship involves not always getting what we want. It's inevitable that in a relationship we have to make some sacrifices – unless we are outrageously rich and famous and can demand compliance from our minions – and most of us are happy to forgo what we want to keep someone we care about happy. But we all have our limits.

In their article 'Giving Up and Giving In: The Costs and Benefits of Daily Sacrifice in Intimate Relationships'[107] Emily Impett et al. look at two competing values in Western society – one that emphasises an ethic of altruism, selflessness, and sacrifice, and the other that emphasises individualism, autonomy, and a relentless pursuit of personal freedom. They make the point that in our intimate relationships, we often find ourselves at a crossroads having to choose between these two paths – giving selflessly to a romantic partner or being true to our own wishes and desires.

For example, a husband has a season ticket for a particular sport that he attends every week. It's an event he loves because he catches up with friends. On request from his wife, he happily stays home from one weekend's game to look after the children so that his wife can meet a friend who has unexpectedly arrived in town. The husband may feel great satisfaction, knowing that he has cared for and responded to his wife in a loving manner. This type of sacrifice moves the husband towards the desired end-state and is called an 'approach motive'.[108] In this scenario, there is no resentment, as the husband willingly gave up his needs for his wife. In contrast, what would happen if the wife had asked her husband to stay home four times during the season, despite knowing the importance of this social activity to her husband and then became very angry and aggressive if he said no? If the husband agrees to stay home to avoid angering his wife or having an argument over the request, he is likely to feel resentment or other negative emotions that detract from his satisfaction in the relationship. This type of sacrifice motivates the husband to avoid an undesired end-state and is called an avoidance motive.

Research has shown that sabotaging or constantly denying your true wishes and desires in a relationship is associated with increased psychological distress and decreased relationship satisfaction. Impett et al. found that those people who sacrificed something because they wanted to avoid an undesirable outcome experienced more negative emotions, lower satisfaction with life, less positive relationship wellbeing, and more relationship conflict. Not a good list of outcomes for anyone, or any relationship.

On the other hand, social psychologists have investigated the positive role sacrifice can play in relationships. There are a variety of demonstrated relational benefits, including increased satisfaction and a greater likelihood of persistence over time to work on overcoming issues. However, findings highlight that it's the motivation for the sacrifice that determines if it will be healthy for the relationship.

Simply put, if your motive for sacrifice is to be loving towards another, then you are more likely to experience a positive outcome. Still, if your motive is to avoid conflict, the long-term consequences will be negative, driven by resentment.

So, what are the wrong reasons to sacrifice your needs for someone else's?

A sacrifice that is motivated by avoidance is going to cause issues in the long run. Conflict avoidance is the main driver for many people who sacrifice their own needs. It might be easier to put up with the snoring than to have a big argument with a partner who resolutely believes a couple should sleep together.

Another misguided motive for sacrifice is the belief that by sacrificing something you want, you will show your partner how much you care for them. You may have had the conversation to explain what is disturbing your sleep, but your partner told you that they just want to be 'close to you' every night, so you continue to endure disturbed sleep to show how much you love them. You may even believe that by sacrificing your own needs, you are providing a good example that your partner will emulate in the future. You may harbour a silent expectation that they will start showing you how much they care for you in return with a sacrifice or two of their own (but they have no idea about this expectation – because you haven't told them). Noble behaviour, but probably futile, and certainly unhealthy.

While the above explains behaviours with seemingly good intentions, it's the motivation behind the sacrifice that makes it unsustainable. If you are left feeling annoyed that you haven't been true to yourself by agreeing to stay in bed with your partner, or you feel that you made the decision to stay there because of an imbalance in power, then we would suggest you consider why you continue to sacrifice your own needs for your partner's needs. Think about what this type of behaviour is achieving in the present and where it is leading as you head into the future.

Yet another misguided reason we sacrifice our needs is to use the sacrifice as a bargaining tool in a future transaction. For example, 'I'll give up my movie night with the girls to go to your last-minute work function if you come to Bill's birthday party with me next week instead of playing golf'. While we have all used this tactic on occasion, if it's an ongoing behaviour in your relationship, it might be time to consider how healthy the dynamics of the relationship are.

Sacrificing your own comfort, pleasure, needs and health for someone else might make you eligible for sainthood, but it's a negotiating technique that relies on an uneven power balance and a degree of disappointment for one person in the relationship. If every time you want pizza you give in and have Thai takeaway to please your partner, we would suggest your partner is not considering your needs and wants. In the long run, is this what you want?

> *Moving to separate rooms was a big plus for us. I was getting to the point where I was really resenting him carrying on with his preferred lifestyle, and I was feeling I just had to go along with it. So now, I am doing what I want to do, and I'm more relaxed. Resentment has been taken out of the equation. I think it's definitely had a beneficial effect.*
> Kaye, 66, together 14 years

If you always agree to have the bedroom temperature at 19°c while you shiver under the sheets, or you give in every night and allow your partner to watch television into the early hours of the morning while you can't sleep, and as a result, you are unhappy and resentful and sleep-deprived, then you aren't being true to yourself or your relationship. If in finding a solution to your sleeping issues, either of you sacrifices something fundamental when you don't really want to avoid conflict, the outcome is again neither sustainable nor beneficial to the relationship. It's not easy.

> *After a year of Greg's snoring getting worse, I decided to start sleeping on the couch in the lounge room. I slept there for about two years. He knew it was happening, but beyond a couple of yelling matches, we only had a bit of a vague, grumbly chat about it. I thought he would offer to go to the couch sometimes or offer to do something about his snoring so I could sleep properly in our bed. Why did I keep doing it? I thought month after month he would see the sacrifice I was making and step up to do something about it. It became a bit of a test I set him – even to see if he would say something, or ask me why I was sleeping out there or if I was getting any sleep. Why didn't I force him to go to the couch? I think I didn't want to hear 'no' as an answer and I really just thought he would do the right thing after seeing what I had done so I could sleep. You think you're leading by example, but in this case, it was my own fault for not speaking up. I'm sure friends probably thought I was being a bit of a martyr and I guess I was. It's separate rooms now though. We finally sorted ourselves out and had a talk about it. I did work it out.*
>
> Maria, 38, database analyst, married 8 years

If you look honestly at your motives for either staying in a disrupted sleeping environment or moving to an alternative sleeping arrangement, and you find that the decision involved a sacrifice you didn't want to make, then it might be back to the drawing board to find another solution that will be longer-lasting, fairer for both of you and better for your relationship.

Compromise

The next level of negotiated outcome is when you and your partner compromise on alternative sleeping arrangements. What's the difference between sacrifice and compromise?

Sacrifice is when one person lets go of something they consider valuable to allow another person to continue to have or do something they want, but the other person does not change at all. Compromise is when you both agree to give up something in exchange for a concession or new behaviour from the other person.

Compromise has greater longevity than sacrifice as a negotiation tool because both parties agree to do (or not do) something for an improved joint outcome. When you are both emotionally or physically invested in a solution, there is a higher chance of success. Compromise still has an element of sacrifice to it as it involves an element of giving up or giving away something as it is a settlement of differences through mutual concession. The significant difference is that both parties are motivated to commit to some type of change to work towards a perceived improvement.

A compromise might be as simple as one person in a couple who wants to sleep together every night, agreeing to let the disturbed sleeper have two nights a week alone in the spare room.

While sacrifice has a win-lose framework, compromise is a little further along the spectrum towards a win-win agreement. However, many argue that because you are both giving something up, it is lose-lose – neither of you gets what you really want. That is relationships though – there is always a need for give and take.

Living with someone is definitely a compromise situation. After 37 years, we decided that we have a spare bed, and whoever feels that they are lacking in a good night sleep can use the spare bed. I always stay up later than my husband (I watch TV or read). He gets up early in the morning (and sneaks out to not wake me).
Kate, www.mamamia.com.au

After the first night I spent with my now husband, he was such a terrible sleeper I told my friends there was no way I could even consider him as a possible boyfriend! To compromise, we now spend maybe two nights per week sleeping apart so we can catch up on sleep and spend the other nights together.
Anonymous, www.mamamia.com

I felt guilty about keeping the light on as it kept him awake. He is such a kind person and considerate of me, so I was happy to turn the light off and not read to be considerate towards him.
Elizabeth, 60, married 25 years

Did we have any feelings of guilt about moving to separate rooms? No. You just get used to it and

accept it. You don't expect the other person to be
perfect. It's just part of the compromise of being
married and putting up with each other's foibles.
Anthony, 62, education professional, married 25 years

When negotiating a compromise, it's important to be clear about what you can and can't accept. This goes back to strong, clear communication. Finding the best compromise may not be one conversation away: it might be twenty discussions away.

My husband and I periodically slept separately,
mainly if we were a bit upset with each other. We
would always end up back in our room together
eventually. After one particular time he left our room
after an argument, I thought really, this is absolutely
heaven. No snoring, I could have the room as I
wanted it with the window open when I wanted it,
and I slept undisturbed by his blanket stealing and
restless sleeping. I still asked him to come back in,
though as I wanted to do the right thing. But when he
had been back in for two days, I thought I don't want
him in here; I don't want to compromise anymore. I
found that so liberating.
Anne, 44, senior manager, married 20 years

About eleven years ago, I started not being able to
sleep because of my husband's snoring. At first, I
would watch a movie on the laptop to drown him out,
but that still meant I couldn't sleep. He's also very
restless and will sometimes hit me, not on purpose
though. Because we don't have a spare room in the

house, I just sleep on the couch now. It's the only
way we are going to stay married because if I had to
sleep in the bed with him, we would be divorced. I
just have a pillow and blanket in the lounge room. I'm
used to it, and I get a much better night's sleep out
there. It's not a failure of our relationship; it's what
works for us. It's what works for me.
Caroline, 30, photographer, married 7 years

Compromise involves change. The industry that has evolved around managing change in humans is enormous. Counsellors, mentors, and self-help gurus recognise the resistance we have to change. We like our lives to be predictable, and when they aren't, we get 'out of whack', don't know what to do and may even start acting out because we are unhappy with the new circumstances in which we find ourselves.

In the context of sleeping, we get used to sleeping on the same side of the bed, sleeping in the same position, with the same pillows and blankets, and in some cases, with the same person next to us. When all our certainty and comfort is challenged, we are likely to feel threatened and defensive and fight to keep what we know, if only because we know it. Keep in mind that with change comes the chance to have a new arrangement that maybe even better than what we had before – we just didn't know it at the time.

Aside from one person moving out of the bed, other types of compromises can take place for bedtime incompatibilities. Solutions such as a person who is disturbed by the light of a reading partner using an eye mask, or the reading partner using an eReader instead of a real book (and a real light), do involve changing our behaviour, but they are small compromises. Other compromises may be more significant.

While not being a huge fan of every technology fad that comes along, I love the iPad. My husband can now read at night without the light having to be on and without the 'swoosh' of the pages turning. He's not allowed to listen to or watch anything on it. It's a good compromise for me needing quiet and a darker room and him wanting to read. Mind you; if it doesn't continue to work, then it's back to the drawing board.
Nicola, 55, retail manager

If I can't sleep, I need to read, and this can sometimes be for a few hours. In those cases, it's me who gets up and goes to the spare room. I know Ann can't sleep if the light is on, so it's not fair to her to do that. Also, if one of us is travelling for work the next day, then the other one has to go to the spare room. This lets the person travelling have access to clothes and the bathroom early in the morning without having to worry about waking the other one. We manage sleeping with a very practical approach.
Neil, 46, HR executive, married 19 years

Our kids are sleeping worse than ever now, and this means that we take turns sleeping between our main room and our spare room. We normally do this night about, but it depends what we have on the next day work-wise. We both want to feel able to cope as much as we can so this means we need to

sleep apart and alternate the good night's sleep with
the broken sleep that comes with looking after the
children. For me, I don't sleep all that well anyway
– and it's getting worse – so having the peace and
quiet of the room downstairs means I have a better
chance of getting a good night's sleep.
Maree, 30, health professional, married 3 years

What will be useful as you work towards finding a compromise is taking the time to really understand your partner's point of view on the situation. If you can take the leap and 'sleep between their sheets' your understanding of what they are agreeing to commit to in the compromise may be more real to you and easier to fit into the context of what you are going to do or give up doing.

Consensus

The third and most successful outcome of a negotiation is reaching consensus.

While compromise still has traces of sacrifice, in that you both make concessions to come to a solution, a consensus is defined as 'solidarity in sentiment and belief', and 'agreement between all the people involved' – for our purposes, all two of you. It's when you can both honestly say, 'I believe this is the best decision we can arrive at for us at this time. I will support what we need to do to make it happen.'

Some argue that a consensus has an element of 'heart' involved over and above the 'head' factor required for compromising. It's when you and your partner can consider all the factors involved in the issue at hand – and that includes each other's perspectives – and come to a decision that you both agree is a solution. A consensus implies a genuine commitment to the decision because both of you have listened to the other's needs and your shared interests have been met. What you have done is looked at the bigger picture of what each of you needs in regard to sleep, considered what's important for both of you and agreed on a new way of 'doing' sleeping at night.

In his book *Consensus Through Conversation*, Larry Dressler[109] highlights why consensus is the most logical and sensible approach to decision making and recommends it when the decision:

- is high-stakes
- has the potential to fragment those involved if made poorly
- involves a solution that will be impossible to implement without strong support and cooperation from those who must implement it
- has no single person who has the ultimate authority to make the decision
- has no single person with all the knowledge required to make the decision
- has people with a stake in the decision having very different perspectives that need to be brought together
- needs a creative solution to address a complex problem.

Although *Consensus Through Conversation* is aimed at a corporate audience, all these descriptors perfectly fit the challenge faced by a couple who can't immediately find a solution that will address the issue of one, or both, of them experiencing sleepless nights.

If you think that there is a grey area between compromise and consensus, you are correct. Consensus involves both of you making changes to your sleeping arrangements. However, it is the attitude towards, and the motivation behind, the decision that takes you from compromise to consensus. It comes down to how you approach the task of finding a solution to the problem and how you accept the solution once it's been agreed upon.

A compromise may see you or your partner holding on to your position, for example, 'I feel like more of a couple when my husband sleeps next to me every night' – but agreeing to behave in a way that doesn't match this. And yet you do it willingly with no resentment, no 'if only …' thoughts. Consensus is about finding a way to shift your thinking, and therefore your position, and work with your partner to find the best solution for both of you.

Most importantly, reaching consensus means that in coming to a decision, neither of you feels that your position on the matter is misunderstood or wasn't heard.

After sleeping apart for a few days, then a few weeks at a time, one night, my wife and I just agreed that the struggle to share a bed wasn't worth it anymore. I resisted the decision most and didn't think I would ever agree to a permanent arrangement of separate rooms. But in the big picture of our lives, it worked best for everyone. I felt a sense of relief, and funnily, really close to her. I still miss having her in the bed

every night but enjoy the times in the early morning
when I slip into her bed and share a few hours
cuddling her. I don't think I will ever feel comfortable
talking about our separate sleeping arrangement as
I think a husband and wife should share a bed, but
my snoring was just too loud. I would rather have my
wife, who sleeps in a separate bed rather than not
have my wife.
Wayne, 41, married 18 years

After 30 years of marriage and many variations on
our sleeping arrangements, sleeping apart was just
so convenient for us both. We are in the same house,
we still see each other, there are as many conjugal
visits as either of us wants, and we both get what we
want from a bedroom. In the big picture, it makes so
much sense. If he wants to come and spend a night,
he can, but he knows that it can't happen too often!
He knows his snoring disturbs me and he cares
enough about me to let me sleep. We've accepted
that this is our sleeping life.
Brooke, 52, educational professional, married 30 years

In trying to reach consensus, you may find a solution that you hadn't thought of before. Consensus involves a degree of 'I have my way of thinking about something, but I could be wrong. So, I am going to listen to you and allow my mind to be influenced by you. I may not fully agree, but hopefully, by sharing and listening, we can agree to a new solution that is ours.' It is an attitude fuelled by goodwill. Remember goodwill?

And while this all sounds warm and fuzzy and oh

so easy, the reality is that it isn't always. If your partner is adamant that you both stay in the same bed because that's what couples do and all you want to do is move into another room because you cannot bear one more hour, let alone night, of their restless legs, then it's going to be tough to find a solution that meets such disparate needs.

Consensus takes time and work. It all depends on where you are coming from and where you are going to. The further apart the positions, the bigger the challenge. This is where you return to the basics of communication and continue to in the hope of finding that elusive and hallowed common ground that just hasn't revealed itself yet.

Humans have an interesting capacity to hear something and go away and ruminate. If a seed of a solution is planted, then the germination time might be a bit longer than you hope but may still take place. So, you may have to sit tight, revisit the topic, and not give up. Onwards and upwards – always.

We talked earlier of the research by Jennifer Hislop about why some women are so readily prepared to sacrifice their own sleep needs for the sake of maintaining a version of how a successful relationship looks.

In reporting her findings, Hislop[110] states that "To sleep apart is to challenge custom, undermine expectations of social order and risk moral censure. Constructing and managing the intimate space of the double bed is thus key to maintaining social order." And that because of this "…couples are prepared to deprioritise their own sleep needs to ensure the maintenance of shared sleeping arrangements and as a symbol of the depth of their loyalty to the relationship. Sleeping together is considered central to the health and well-being of the relationship; a morally right 'thing to do'; part of the marriage contract; and a behavioural pattern passed down from parent to child over the generations".

It is important to notice that, as described above, sleeping together is merely a modern-day, western, social construct rather than the biological/physiological norm. One result of this perception of sleeping together as normal and the right thing to do.

Hislop and Arber 2003[111] found that women prioritise their partner's sleep above their own even to the extent where a woman's "concern for her partner's well-being may include responsibility for his sleep, inciting feelings of guilt if she inadvertently disturbs this sleep".

This necessarily implies that women are sacrificing, or at least compromising, their sleep to ensure that their, male, partner gets good sleep and even feel guilty when they disturb their sleep. In practice this could mean that they modify their behaviour in various ways, e.g., laying still when they are awake in the night, not getting up to go to the bathroom etc.

It would seem that women sacrifice their sleep and their physical and emotional well-being because society has convinced them of the 'normality' of sleeping together and because of this 'normality' they find it so hard to consider the idea of sleeping apart.

Can't get to yes?

After you and your partner have demonstrated outstanding communication skills, and you've both showered each other in boundless goodwill to find a solution to your sleeping issues, then what next? We'll get to that in the next couple of chapters. First, we want to talk about what happens when you don't reach an agreement.

Sometimes the best-laid plans don't turn out as expected. Sometimes it's not until the twenty-fourth revision that you manage to get it right. You both need to retain flexibility while you determine what works for you and keep talking. Don't stop talking. If you haven't been great communicators in the past, this could be a chance for both of you to hone your skills and rediscover a genuine interest in each other.

Be honest with each other about what is working and what is not. There is a chance that you will have adjustments to make that create tension and friction as you iron out the details, but honesty communication should help you over any rough patches.

What if all your attempts at trying to renegotiate your sleeping arrangements don't work? Even with all the will and best intentions in the world, you and your partner may not be able to find a solution that suits you both, and that is a tough place to be.

John Gottman, psychologist and researcher who runs *The Love Lab*,[112] says that he can predict how long a couple will last, not by studying how well a couple gets along, but by studying how well a couple doesn't get along. He notes that a relationship is only as strong as its weakest moments; these surface when a couple faces tough challenges.

As hard as it is to accept, some problems don't have solutions. The reality for some couples is that sleeping issues may cause, or be a significant contributor to, the end of a relationship.

My relationship ended because my partner could not
accept that I wanted to sleep in a separate room.
No matter how much I explained the substantial
impact on my health from not sleeping, he would
sit on the chair in the bedroom and say 'we've got
to get this right because if we don't get it right, the
relationship's finished'. His mother had dealt with her
inability to sleep by taking sleeping pills, and he was
set in his ways about what a traditional relationship
looked like – two people sharing a bed. I tried to
explain that our relationship didn't need to end
just because I needed to sleep in a bed by myself
every night. A couple of weeks after I told him I was
moving into a separate room, our relationship ended.
Louise, 48, teacher

If you can't find a solution with your partner to your sleeping issues, the best advice we can give is to keep trying. By this, we don't mean that you should keep trying the *same* thing repeatedly. That just makes you eligible for insanity by Albert Einstein's definition: 'Doing the same thing over and over again and expecting a different result'. But you also need to remember Winston Churchill's equally worthy advice: 'Never, never, never, give up'.

If your solution isn't working, you will need to try something different, such as:

- Finding other couples who sleep apart (there are lots out there once you start asking around) that your partner would trust and ask them how they make it work.
- Trying different ways of finding out your partner's

motivations for staying in the same bed and working to ease their fears that the practice threatens your relationship.

- Finding a less dramatic solution than moving to separate rooms by suggesting small adjustments to your partner, thereby letting them work through the change in a way that is not as confronting.
- Making sure the topic doesn't disappear off your relationship radar by continuing to refer to it or taking the chance to talk about the effects of sleep deprivation, etc. (this may be interpreted as nagging, but it is all in the delivery).

If all your efforts do not bring about a successful resolution that both of you can live with, you may need to consider external help in the form of a counsellor. Whatever you do, if it's imperative to you, don't give up.

Pause for thought…

- Have you ever analysed the process you follow to resolve conflict, and if you have, does it work or could it do with some improvements?
- Is one of you more of a peacemaker than the other?
- Is one of you more inclined to sacrifice your needs for the other?
- What happens when you come to an impasse on other issues? How do you resolve these situations?
- Can you think of a situation where you have

reached a compromise or consensus? What did that look like for both of you, and how did you get there?

- Are you individually, or as a couple, capable of talking to other people – parents or friends – to see if they have solutions you can't see?
- Would you consider seeking help from a counsellor to work through issues that you are not able to resolve yourselves?

SIX

How to make sleeping separately work

The best laid schemes o' mice an' men
Often go awry
And leave us nothing but grief and pain
For promised joy.
Robert Burns (1785)[113]

We all love that spine-tingling moment when a wave of brilliance arrives to resolve a problem, and we make a plan. We organise our resources, rally the troops, communicate the plan to all involved and remind ourselves why we rule the world and are masters of our destiny.

The tricky thing about a plan is that it's just that – a plan; a proposed and sometimes inaccurate prediction about how something will be in the future. One of Jennifer's 'go to' sayings is a version of wise words from

Moltke the Edler, a German field marshal who said words to the effect of 'a plan rarely survives contact with reality'. A plan is a course of action you think will bring about an intended and hopefully beneficial outcome. But life is unpredictable, and worse still, so are the other people whose help you often need to execute your plan. How many great projects have you made that have been ruined by bad weather, a late bus, a lost friend or a person who cancels on you at the last minute?

Still, our indefatigable spirit means that we never stop making plans, which is good. If we did stop, we would never solve problems, launch into exhilarating adventures, or go to fantastic dinner parties with friends.

Once you and your partner decide that your sleeping arrangements need to change, then it's time for you both to put your heads down and plan. As someone once said[114]: 'The best way to predict the future is to invent it' to which can be added a quote from Alan Lakein. a well-known author on personal time management, said "Planning is bringing the future into the present so that you can do something about it now." Planning gives you a sense of control by working towards making the unknown known. The question is: what is your plan and what factors do you include when sitting down to decide the fate of your slumbering future?

For some couples, a change in sleeping arrangements just happens. An unspoken understanding that sees one person move to another room because of disturbed sleep that results in a permanent move that is never discussed or formally agreed. Even though some couples can work within the framework of an unspoken agreement, such arrangements can be a *Titanic* heading out to sea.

When my husband started sleeping in the lounge room, it just kind of happened. He liked watching sport on TV, so would often sleep on a mattress in the lounge as I didn't like TV in the bedroom. There was no discussion; it was just convenient for both of us. When the kids left home, he moved into his own bedroom, where he now has a TV. We weren't upset about the arrangement, so I guess we didn't feel like we had to talk about it. We talk about a lot of other things in our marriage but just didn't talk about sleeping separately.
Brooke, 52, educational consultant, married 30 years

The decision to sleep apart happened gradually. We lasted one year in a bed together after we were married, but even in that first year his snoring was so loud, I would regularly disappear during the night to another room. Over time, I started disappearing more and more during the night, but he was such a heavy sleeper that he didn't notice. There was no specific discussion where we sat down, but I think there was an understanding about why I was leaving.
Leanne, 41, HR executive, married 15 years

One day it dawned on me that he hadn't come to bed for quite a few months. He wasn't cold-shouldering me, and there was no attitude, but I realised we weren't sleeping together anymore. There was no specific discussion, but we did have a conversation one day that unless his snoring stopped, we would probably never sleep together again.
Suzette, 40, administrative assistant, married 17 years

We never made a formal decision to sleep separately.
How it went was I would sleep at his place sometimes
when we weren't living together, and then he would
learn that I got grumpy after not sleeping that well.
Then I would kind of do both when we were living
together but did have my own room when we first
got a place together. I definitely slept in the same bed
more frequently back then because I wanted to show
I was trying, but the quality of sleep never improved.
Now, I try less because we have a child, are so much
busier, and the sleep quality is that much more
important. I definitely think formally discussing it is the
way to go because there are a lot of emotions around
it that keep continuing when you don't talk about it
directly. If you just do it at the beginning and have
a plan, there is less negative emotion. For instance,
whenever we would get into a big argument about
something, my husband would bring this up and then
I would feel crummy all over again. 'You haven't been
trying; etc.' because we never defined the parameters,
to begin with. If you leave things 'open' then there
is miscommunication and misunderstanding and a
whole wack of negative emotions that come with it.
So therefore, I would far more prefer some negative
emotion up front but a concrete plan/decision that is
worked on in the beginning.
Christine, 35, working mother, married 10 years

Jennifer knows that if she and her husband hadn't talked
about the decision to sleep separately, she would have
had a hundred questions floating around in her head.
And in the absence of answers from her husband, would

have made them up. Even though she knew that sleeping together wasn't an option for them, she still needed to know answers to some practical questions when they moved to their separate rooms, such as:

- Would her husband still want to kiss and cuddle her?
- Would they still have a sex life?
- How did her husband feel about sleeping separately?
- How would they tell people about our decision?
- Could either of them go to the other person's bed if they wanted?
- Jennifer also needed some fairly silly questions answered too:
- Would her husband miss her at night?
- Would he think less of her or our relationship because they were in different rooms?

Jennifer is happy to admit that she is not very composed when she has unanswered questions hovering in her mind. While she doesn't mind answers she may not like, she would much prefer an answer that is 'no' to no answer at all. Left alone, she admits that her brain is too creative and often errs on the negative. Neil's experience was somewhat different as his irregular schedule meant that it was easy for his partner to understand the benefits of sleeping separately from the start. While there was some concern that his partner was not altogether happy to sleep separately, it only took the occasional one night sleeping together to remove any doubt about it being the right way to go.

Planning to change your sleeping arrangements can

range from having a quick, light-hearted, and amicable chat, to an in-depth and confronting discussion that lasts for hours (or days) through to documenting your decisions, so you have something to refer back to if details are forgotten in the future. The nature and seriousness of the discussion and planning will depend on how you best like to work when making joint decisions. If your plan is very detailed, capturing it on paper is a good idea. This could help avoid the 'but remember you said you would move to the spare room if you woke me two times in a row, not three' type of arguments. We would recommend that if there are metrics or a level of detail in what you are planning, then as a minimum, jot a few points down that you both agree to – but refrain from having it witnessed by a court officer!

If you are making a purposeful decision to change your sleeping arrangements, even a brief discussion will help create the space to bring in the changes. It will alert both you and your partner to the fact that life in bed is going to be different and might avoid the situation where one of you feels as though the other has engaged in a covert operation designed to un-nerve or un-hinge you through deceptive bedtime behaviour. Whether planning a brief discussion or a major diplomatic offensive, remember the framework from Chapter four and answer the questions how, why, when, where and what.

Also, as discussed in Chapter four, it is a wise idea to consider a range of options when deciding how your sleeping arrangements are going to change. There are many variations of the theme of sleeping apart and although having completely separate bedrooms is as far away from sleeping together as you can get (without heading to separate houses – although that's an option that more and more people are considering and opting for – see www.apartners.com for some information about this quickly growing domestic arrangement), there are many possibilities between these two ends of the spectrum.

Importantly, be open to the likelihood that the first change you make to your sleeping arrangements may not be the last. Like many facets of your relationship, sleeping arrangements evolve and may need tweaking and tuning to get them right.

Klösch[115] says that "sleeping as a pair is not a fixed system that has to remain constant for years or decades once it has been established … sleeping is a dynamic process influenced by many different factors such as age, gender, degree of stress, day of the week and even weather condition". In itself, the process of ageing and maturing precipitates ongoing change. Few people have the same haircut or wear the same fashion as they sported a decade ago. So just as you accept that low-slung jeans or skimpy tops no longer flatter your developing mid-section, decisions you make now about sleeping arrangements may not suit you in a year or a decade. What's great about being a grown-up is that we can change our minds and try new things all the time – with the cooperation of and in consultation with our partner, of course.

When you begin your planning phase, be mindful of the emotional responses that talking about the changes such as nightly separation might have on you. If you are up to it, name your emotions as they surface, both positive and negative. Ask your partner how they feel as you talk about your plans. For example, 'I think I'm going to feel really sad and a bit guilty the first night I go to bed in the spare room. How do you think you will feel?' or 'I appreciate and am grateful that you understand how I feel about not having the TV on in the bedroom, and I know you are giving up something you really enjoy so I can sleep better'.

The suggestions we make are by no means comprehensive. Hopefully, some of them might be what you are looking for, while others might spark an idea for a solution to your particular sleeping problem.

To clarify what we mean by 'alternative sleeping arrangements', we mean an alternative to a traditional couple's sleeping arrangement where most resources in the main bedroom are shared, and both of you climb into the same bed every night, share bedding, and wake up together every morning.

We group the range of alternative sleeping arrangements under three headings:

- The paddling pool
- The wading pool
- Diving into the deep end.

The paddling pool

Offering solutions that don't actually involve either of you moving to a separate room might seem contrary to the spirit of this book, but, if you are at the stage where you and your partner don't need to, or cannot bear the thought of, sleeping in separate rooms, there are steps you can take that allow you to splash around in the paddling pool of alternative sleeping arrangements. Depending on what your bedroom issues are, you may start to find relief for your ills by changing some of the physical aspects of your bedroom or the behavioural aspects of the people who sleep in it.

Just remember that separate sleeping is not for everyone – but getting a good night's sleep is.

Even making small changes to your current sleeping and bedroom behaviours may pave the way towards a better night's sleep.

Bedtime stories

In the battle of 'the bed readers vs the bed sleepers', there are several behavioural and environmental changes you can make that will let both of you have your needs met.

- The person who likes to read could stay in the lounge to read rather than reading in bed.
- You could negotiate a specific amount of time for reading in bed – e.g., half an hour.
- The reader could buy an e-Reader to minimise the noise from turning pages and, if the light from the eReader is a problem, negotiate a level of brightness with which you can both live.
- The reader could buy a book light that fits directly over the book to minimise light in the room.
- One or both of you could investigate bedside lights that give a more focused beam of light.
- The sleeper could wear an eye mask until the reader is ready to turn the light out.

*Oh, my boyfriend and I have had some fun
negotiating this one. I absolutely must read before I
sleep, and if the book is good, I can read for a couple
of hours before I even know it. He insists that the
bedside light has to be off so he can sleep, so I've
settled on reading by candlelight. I have a candle
in a big hurricane lamp, which works fine for me. It
actually feels sort of cozy, especially in winter. The
trick, of course, is to be sure to blow it out before
you fall asleep!*
Rohanna, 25, student

*One word – Kindle. All the fighting, all the tossing
and turning and 'humphing' disappeared in an
instant. It was a miracle.*
Lisa, 45, mother of two, married 25 years

*Little lamps and eye masks don't work for my
husband or me. Either we both stay awake with lights
on in bed, or we both sleep with lights off in bed. If
one of us can't sleep and the other one must sleep,
then the one who can't sleep leaves the bedroom.
When we're at a motel, I sit in the bathroom to read.*
Elaine, 48, married 22 years

Old bed, hard bed, soft bed … new bed?

The age and suitability of the bed you share may be
the cause of your sleeping problems. If you have been
sleeping on the same old mattress, on the same old
frame for a long, long time, you might benefit from an
upgrade. Many factors can impact on mattress comfort

for couples, and differing needs in style and firmness of mattresses become more common as people age.

Bad backs, hips, shoulders, and necks can legitimately lead to couples needing mattresses that have different levels of firmness. The most common way to solve this is to change your bed to one that accommodates two different levels of firmness. This could be one mattress with differing levels of firmness on each side or two single beds that can be put together to form one king-size bed. A quick search on the internet will provide you with the information you need. This solution may see you heading to the Manchester department to purchase new bed linen, so dust off your credit card in preparation.

If you must deal with a restless sleeper, you may need a new mattress that minimises the impact of their movement on you. Latex mattresses offer this feature and might be just what you are looking for. Again, a couple of hours on the internet might prove to be an enlightening experience. If you prefer face-to-face research, a discussion about your sleep issues with a bed salesperson will update you on the available possibilities.

Maybe you just need to consider a bigger bed? Two couples Jennifer knows – both in their mid-forties – still sleep in double beds. Jennifer is amazed that they can find the comfort necessary to sleep each night, but they do and speak fondly of enjoying their cosy environment. Many couples find that by moving to a king-size, or super king-sized bed, they have enough space to escape a heavy breathing or restless partner. This size of bed also accommodates those who like to exercise creativity in their sleeping positions throughout the night. If you have ever slept in a super king-sized bed, you will know that the challenge is sometimes finding the other person, rather than being disturbed by them.

Recently we purchased a king-size bed. It's great, and the tossing, turning and snoring are not so bad now. I am sure it's due to the extra space under the covers. I find it also romantic reaching out whilst under the covers of a big bed and touching and caressing the one I love. My husband agrees.
MM, www.radionational.com.au/lifematters

Temperature tantrums

Research shows that the ideal temperature range for sleeping differs widely for each person. The wide fluctuations mean that there is no prescribed best room temperature to produce optimal sleep patterns. We simply sleep best at the temperature that feels most comfortable to each of us – just the same as some of us enjoy living in the tropics and some of us love arctic climates. (Another question to add to your speed-dating checklist.)

That said, extreme temperatures in sleeping environments do disrupt sleep.[116] REM sleep, which we know is one of the critical deep sleep phases, is more sensitive to temperature-related disruption. For example, in freezing temperatures, we can be entirely deprived of REM sleep, so a complaint about being too hot or too cold to sleep is legitimate. What can you do?

If the temperature difference is minor, you can investigate quilts that are weighted differently on each side. Similarly, having separate quilts, blankets and sheets will allow each of you to sleep at your ideal temperature.

Having central heating in the house means that my wife is able to have the bedroom quite warm. When I then have to sleep under a thick quilt, I end up throwing it off every night, but then wake up periodically a little chilly, then hot again after the quilt goes back on, then hot, etc. etc. I could have slapped myself across the back of the head for not thinking of separate quilts sooner. Such an obvious and simple solution. Now I just have to get her to turn the TV off.
Francis, 37, engineer, married 7 years

I have always slept with my sheets tucked in so was frequently annoyed when my husband insisted on having his feet out every night to sleep as he complained the bed was too warm and having his feet out regulated his temperature. He would even do it in winter. I know it probably sounds very petty, but it annoyed me to think that the sheets were untucked on the other side of the bed, and I would sometimes lie awake and think about it. After discussing it with a sympathetic friend, I cut all our sheets up the middle to halfway and now wrap the side in the middle of the bed round my feet. Problem solved. I'm really quite normal otherwise.
Milly, 52, married 30 years

Fans and air conditioning are areas of potentially tough negotiation. When one person can't sleep with a fan or air conditioner on, and the other can't sleep without it, it is a challenging situation. Consensus may be impossible; compromise is likely to leave both parties still giving up something they may need to sleep properly and sacrifice, well, we know where that ends.

Some problems don't have a solution. Many people I interviewed cited extreme temperature differences as the cause of sleeping separately. No paddling pool for them.

Bedtime

If you have issues around what time you go to bed at night and get up in the morning, you may need to give your creativity a good work out in devising solutions around how you to avoid waking each other up. As we know that forcing a change on your body clock is not going to work, you may have to accept that this is going to be a long-term challenge.

Some suggestions to get you going:

- Lay rugs or runners on a wooden floor to help to minimise the disturbance of a noisy walker.
- Agree that when the lark heads off to bed, the owl gets ready as well, but doesn't actually go to bed until later.
- Use a low-illumination night light for the owl's convenience when they do come to bed.
- Agree that the lark's gear for the next day will be readily available in another part of the house, so no raking through the wardrobe and drawers takes place in the morning.

Would you stop that!

As we discussed in chapter three, there is a range of annoying behaviours that you can try to limit through intervention if you want to sleep together, such as snoring, stealing sheets and blankets, using laptops, watching television, grinding teeth and breathing noisily.

For example, agree on such arrangements as:

- After the first/second/third/nth time that your partner's snoring wakes you, you are allowed to awaken them to change position (irrespective of whether they agree they were snoring or not).
- If retrieving your stolen sheets wakes the 'thief', then that's the price they have to pay for taking them in the first place.
- If your partner has moved such that their breathing or teeth grinding wakes you, you are allowed to do what is needed to make them roll away to minimise the noise.

This story from the *Wall Street Journal*[117] may provide you with a workable process…

> *Rochelle Thomas has gotten so fed up with her husband's snoring over the years that she's created a 'three strikes rule.' Each time he wakes her up with his snorts, honks or shudders – shaking the mattress 'like a cheap motel-bed vibrator' – she gives him a penalty.*
> *Strike one: A nudge.*

Strike two: A shove or kick.

Strike three: He's out – of the bed and down the hall to the guest room.

'It prevents anger in the morning from lack of sleep,' says Ms. Thomas, a sales representative from La Mirada, Calif. 'And I think it just may have saved his life, because I am sure I would have killed him by now.'

Similarly, if one of you has needs that impact on the other because you are getting out of bed at times or with a frequency that disturbs the other's sleep, then alternative arrangements might minimise the disruption – depending on the facilities in your house:

- If your partner's use of the ensuite toilet at night-time wakes you, ask them to use another toilet.
- If you have only one bathroom in the house and it's so close to the room that its use during the night wakes the sleeper, agree not to turn the lights on or flush the toilet if it is used just for urinating.
- If one of you has to get up early for work, or sport, or anything, then all clothes, accessories, etc. that are needed are taken out the night before and put somewhere else in the house, and another bathroom (if available) is used to get ready.
- If one of you is always later to bed than the other, then lights are not turned on, and the ensuite is not used for teeth cleaning or before-bed toileting (again, if another bathroom is available).

When it comes to appliances in the bedroom, there needs to be some give and take if you want to continue sharing a bed. My best suggestion is that the times for use are negotiated. For example, television viewing only until 11 pm, or laptop used only for 30 minutes after going to bed. This will definitely be a situation of compromise, so all the best on this particular negotiation.

Miscellany

There are several other practical solutions for the parade of bedroom problems. Here are some suggestions for dealing with some of the other issues we have identified.

- If one person is bothered by a partner who prefers to sleep in the nude, then the nude partner is not allowed to touch the clothes wearer during the night unless permission is granted; if naked sleepers want to cuddle, they need to consider wearing PJs.
- If one partner cannot sleep if there is light in the room, invest in a comfortable and effective eye mask.
- If noise is keeping one partner awake, investigate the range of earplugs on the market or look into purchasing a white-noise or sound machine to create a constant background distraction.
- If eating is leaving a mess in the bed and the bedroom, agree that only certain types of food be allowed in the room and that a 'no plates in

the bedroom' rule applies so all dishes must go back to the kitchen before lights out.

- If children in the bed are squeezing one or both of you out, take some time to re-negotiate boundaries with your children and/or spouse about sleeping and bedrooms.
- If pets are causing a nightly exodus, you can invest in a pet bed for the bedroom.
- If the occasional illness is an issue, for example, during cold and 'flu season, pre-negotiate an agreement that one of you will temporarily relocate for a period of time, so you don't have to try to negotiate such matters at 2 am.

The suggestions above are in no way exhaustive, but hopefully provide some examples of what might be negotiated to address common disturbances. Your particular situation may require a variation on one of the above suggestions. If your dilemma is not explicitly answered, we hope there is something in this chapter that gets your creative juices flowing. We don't have, and nor do we think there is, a silver bullet for everyone's unique sleeping dilemma.

The priority is to focus on a solution and not the problem, keep talking and don't limit your thinking to the obvious. Ask yourself this question: 'What needs to be different to make this work?' and revisit the idea of brainstorming solutions. The most sensible idea might come out of the most ridiculous suggestion.

If none of these ideas sounds like the solution you are after, or you have come back to the book because you have tried several solutions but still aren't getting the night's sleep you know you deserve, then it might be time to graduate from the paddling pool to the wading pool.

The wading pool

If you know that you are unable to spend every night in the same bed and/or the same room as your partner, then there are many options to investigate. Again, keeping an open mind and thinking outside the box will help you find the answer to your problems.

Many couples find the answer to sleeplessness comes in the form of having semi-permanent arrangements to sleep apart. These types of arrangements are very common for couples that realise they have an issue sleeping together that cannot be resolved, but still want to spend some nights in bed together when it suits them. They like the idea of sharing a common bedroom, but value and need their sleep enough to sleep apart sometimes. How often this part-time arrangement is used, of course, depends on the issues and needs of each couple.

Some of these arrangements could be:

- Agreeing to sleep in the spare room sometimes – you can negotiate the number of times you use the spare room option, who goes to the spare room and the reasons why one of you goes there.
- If there is no spare room available, have a mattress (comfortable and pre-made) available in another room such as a study or children's room for nights when separation is needed.

- Buy a sofa bed for a study or sunroom and make sure it is pre-made and ready for full- or part-night use.
- If the situation is desperate, agree on a set of circumstances that might lead to one of you sleeping on the couch sometimes. If this happens often enough, have a set of bed linen (pillow, sheet, duvet/blanket) ready and easily accessible for the bedroom refugee to take to the couch.

Another advantage of using a spare room for occasional sleeping is the continuing relationship that is maintained within the main bedroom. This relationship allows couples to keep connected using the main room as a base and just sleep elsewhere. Some might argue this is semantic – but try telling that to the couples who have found their sleeping nirvana in this arrangement.

We call our spare room the 'sleep sanctuary'. Whoever really needs to sleep is allowed to spend the night there. Juggling careers and two young children means that there are months when we don't sleep together in the bed in our room because one of us is in the 'sleep sanctuary', but we choose sleep over being in the same bed at this point in our lives. If we are on holidays, then we have no issue being in the same bed – but when it's our normal life, sleep is essential.
Maree, 30, health professional, married 3 years

We have a spare room that one of us will sleep in maybe 2–3 times a week. Often the discussion

*about who will sleep there happens just before we
go to bed. If he is travelling, I find out what time he
is getting up, and I will decide to go to the other
bed if it's going to be so early that it will disturb my
sleep. We mainly start in the same bed each night if
one of us isn't travelling. But if I can't sleep – which
happens a bit – I like to read. This disturbs Ann,
so I get up and go to the spare room. It takes the
pressure off both of us, and we both sleep better. It's
simply a practical solution that lets us get the sleep
we need to deal with life.*
Ann and Neil, both 46, HR executives, married 19 years

*I only started using the spare room to sleep when I
read an article about it at the beginning of the year.
Neither of us had thought about it before – we just
thought it was a traditional thing to sleep with each
other every night. We both sleep so much better in
separate rooms; it's definitely been of benefit to both
of us. But where I sleep is still just the spare room – I
haven't slept between the sheets yet, just under the
quilt cover and on the top sheet. My pyjamas are still
under the pillow of our bed in our room, I get ready
for bed every night in our room, and I walk right
past a bathroom to use the ensuite in our room. Our
bedroom is still a part of me; I just don't sleep there
every night anymore.*
Elizabeth, 60, married 25 years

Another arrangement that might work for couples that
are dealing with a restless partner is to have separate
beds in the same room. Depending on the size of your

bedroom and available funds, it could be feasible to have two double beds or two super-single beds in the same room. Hopping into your partner's bed for a quick cuddle will undoubtedly be easier and nighttime and morning chats will be unhindered.

If you know that you are neither a paddler nor a wader because you have tried some of these fixes with no success, or you just know that it's time to make the break and have your own room, then let's look at what's involved in diving into the deep end and really sleeping apart.

Diving into the deep end

Explaining the technical part of this arrangement is easy. You and your partner sleep separately every night.

In the deep end, you and your partner have separate rooms, or one of you sleeps in a different part of the house every night, but you still share the amenities of the main bedroom.

Sleeping apart permanently comes to some couples slowly. A traditional – or normal – start to a relationship or marriage sees most couples sharing a bed quite happily, but factors such as snoring, illness, children or changing priorities see them deciding at some point that separate rooms are the best.

We started sleeping together at the beginning of the marriage, but he was younger, thinner and didn't snore as loudly. Right from the beginning, I did need earplugs, though. He comes from a family of snorers,

*and his parents have slept separately for the last 25
years.*
Suzette, 40, administrative assistant, married 17 years

*We slept together for quite a while at the beginning.
Doug started falling asleep on the couch, and I
tended to leave him there as his snoring was getting
worse, and if I woke him and made him come
through to bed, I would be the one who was kept
awake because of his snoring. This lasted until about
four years ago when we finally agreed that separate
rooms were the best arrangement for us.*
Penny, 40, mother, married 14 years

*In the beginning, we were very old fashioned and
'didn't do that' (sleep apart). I started working in
the bedding department of Myer in the 1980s and
was shocked to find out that married couples slept
in separate beds. I thought there must have been
a problem in their marriage. But over the last 15
years, I started to snore, John's hearing became very
delicate, and he started to not sleep as deeply. I also
like listening to the radio when I go to bed, and that
would drive him mad. I tried a few things to stop my
snoring, like making a band out of t-shirt ribbing that I
put around my jaw, but nothing worked, and we were
getting less and less sleep. You have to adapt as you
change and get older, so I shifted to the spare room.*
May, 66, retired, married 40 years

*Margaret started working night shifts, so she was
getting home at about 2 am, but not being ready for*

bed until about 4.30 am. This meant she would wake me up about an hour before I would normally get up. I know she was complaining that I would thrash around in the bed a lot – she says I'm 'theatrical in bed' – and apparently I snore. Anyway, I was losing sleep because of her sleep patterns so a few years ago we agreed that it would be best if she moved to the bedroom downstairs. We're both very happy with the decision.
John, 58, building contractor, married 30 years

For us, we ended up in separate rooms for a few reasons. Probably because I had a lot of surgery, then he got his knee operated on, and I thought I deserved a bit of room to myself. After I had spent some time in a bedroom by myself because of my surgery, I realised how good it was having your own space. There was no going back. When we have to share a bed now, it's awful.
Von, 72, married 55 years

For other couples, the decision to sleep apart happens pretty darn quickly, though this is less common than those who find it becomes a necessity over time.

Michael and I met at 14, married six years later and have never been able to sleep together. We thought we would just get married and start sleeping with each other – but it didn't happen. We tried to sleep in the same bed, but one of us always ended up in the spare bed. We were both reasonably relaxed about it right from the beginning. It never caused a big issue

for us. The bigger issue was the frustration of not being able to sleep so the decision to finally have separate rooms was liberating.
Melissa, 47, executive, married 27 years

If your planning leads you to decide that you are moving to sleep separately, then there are several sub-plans that need to be made.

Where are you going to sleep?

If there is an available spare room in your house, then you are set. The question you will need to address is who is moving to the spare room? This one might be tricky if the bedroom you currently share is bigger, has an ensuite, has air-conditioning, has all the closet space, favourite furniture, etc. How are you going to decide who moves and who gets to stay? Flip a coin? Paper-scissors-rock? It could prove to be a tough decision.

Jennifer's husband's bedroom is much larger than hers and has an ensuite. It's certainly the pick of the two bedrooms, but she prefers her room because of its positioning to catch the night-time breezes in summer, and she did not want to give them up – so they had an easy task negotiating who slept where.

If one of you is more eager to move to another room than the other, then that person may find they are the one taking the less-well-appointed room, but this is not a given. It's all about negotiating what's best for both of you, given your own particular circumstances.

For couples who have children or extended families, a spare room is a rare commodity. This creates a substantial problem that needs to be factored into any plans. This particular challenge is most commonly solved by the use of the humble, but trusty, couch.

After my time sleeping on the couch, we decided that I would permanently move to a separate room. Unfortunately, there was only a small spare room towards the back of the house, near the kitchen. As much as I hated to admit it, I knew that that's where I was going because I was the one making all the fuss about Greg keeping me from sleeping. However, I am very happy to say that after a bit of whinging on my part, we renovated the room, which involved investing in some good carpet and a very quiet reverse-cycle air conditioner. I have a great bed, even though it's just a double, with very nice bed linen. And when I need a glass of water in the night, it's just a short walk.
Maria, 38, database analyst, married 8 years

When we came to the agreement that we were no longer going to be able to share a bed successfully, we figured it was easier for him to just stay sleeping on the couch. We don't have a spare room because we have children and a house that just fits us all, so we bought a really comfortable couch that he can totally stretch out on and sleep. It's a proper single-bed-sized couch, and that was our compromise. The good thing is that this is only a temporary solution as we are building another room for him next year. Seeing as he has the most trouble getting

to, and staying asleep, being on the couch means
that he can watch TV when he wakes at night.
Suzette, 40, administrative assistant, married 17 years

I have been with my husband for 13 years, but for the
past 11, we have had trouble sharing a bed. Because
of space problems in the house due to number of
people vs number of rooms, I sleep on the couch.
Sleeping there doesn't affect my health; a lack of
sleep does though. It happened over time. I got
sick to death of getting out of bed and going to the
couch, so now I just have a pillow and blanket out
there all the time.
Caroline, 30, photographer, married 7 years

Re-negotiating the romance

This section may also be relevant to those who are in the wading pool but wading in deeper and deeper and spending more nights apart than together. Keeping connected to your partner through intimate behaviour is important when you aren't sleeping in the same bed every night. It's what makes your relationship different from the other relationships in your life. As we have mentioned several times, we are not talking just about sex. While that's important, it's the smaller acts of intimacy that can be forgotten or put in the too-hard basket when you don't have the daily chance to connect emotionally, socially, and physically in bed together.

Dr Timothy Sharp, Clinical and Coaching Psychologist and founder of the Happiness Institute,[118] says that couples should think about the constructs of intimacy as it relates to them as a couple. He emphasises that intimacy and sleep are separate. 'It's important to understand the separation, and then it's important to think what intimacy actually is for you. Intimacy can occur at different levels and in many different ways. Yes, part of intimacy is sexual intercourse, and other physical acts, but they can be done in many locations at any time of the day. Then there are other parts of intimacy, hugging, holding hands, kissing, that can also be done at any time of the day and anywhere. I would encourage couples to define intimacy as broadly as possible and not limit it to just sex in bed at night. Intimacy can be whatever you want it to be, in different ways and different times. If you choose to sleep separately, it does not mean you have not chosen to be intimate.'

On the flip side, though, just because you move to separate rooms does not mean you suddenly have to become a couple who kisses and cuddles every time you see each other in the kitchen. What is most important is that neither of you feels as though you have lost too much intimacy because of the sleeping choices you have made.

Dr Barbara Bartlik,[119] a New York psychiatrist and sex therapist, has identified the three most significant challenges couples face when they decide to sleep apart. While recognising that 'sleeping soundly benefits people on all levels, mind and body, and directly contributes to a longer and happier life', she also makes the point that couples in this situation should 'institute strategies and rituals focused on keeping them connected romantically rather than just living together as companionable housemates'.

Dr Bartlik's challenges and solutions are:

- **Less loving touch:** Even when couples aren't accustomed to holding one another all night long, a lot of touching goes on while falling asleep and during the night. Whether intentional or not, touch enhances intimacy. It also has a measurable biological effect, stimulating oxytocin, the hormone that promotes a sense of bonding.

  The solution: Dr Bartlik urges couples to make a concerted effort to stay touchy-feely during the day. Don't just walk by each other—stop for a casual kiss or a loving pat. Hold hands on the couch, and cuddle while you watch TV.

- **No opportunity for pillow talk:** You may have lots of focused conversations about the children, the car, and the dog, but there's something uniquely intimate in the kind of pillow talk that meanders here and there as you're relaxing and readying yourself to doze off at night or as you awaken and get set to take on the day. Good marriages thrive on these private, unplanned, and uninterrupted conversations.

  The solution – a hybrid arrangement: Dr Bartlik suggests trying to fall asleep in the same bed but with the agreement that if one partner's night-time habits interrupt the other's sleep, it's perfectly okay for him/her to slip off to go sleep in a different room – then toward morning, the one who wakes up first can slip into bed with the other to share those close first few minutes of your day.

- **Fewer sexual interludes:** Not surprisingly, diminished sexual intimacy is the greatest concern people have about sleeping apart, but Dr Bartlik says that she knows many couples whose sex lives are enhanced by separate rooms – it can even lead to greater desire! This makes sense for several reasons: research shows that being sleep-deprived lowers testosterone in both men and women, which interferes with sexual desire for both genders and also makes it harder for men to have an erection and women to achieve orgasm. In Dr Bartlik's view, this is a more significant threat to intimacy than just the fact of sleeping separately. And there's also the fact that absence can, indeed, make the heart – and other body parts – grow fonder. You know what I mean.

The solution: Getting more rest will almost certainly help boost your libido. Therefore, she suggests that couples that sleep apart should make a special point of having sex regularly. If the idea of a scheduled 'date night' sounds unromantic to you, why not approach it in a way that adds sizzle to your sex life? Try to establish romantic rituals that bring you close, such as sending sexy notes to each other, lighting candles for dinner or taking a bath together. You can also make a point of engaging in pleasurable but not sexual activities that include touch such as dancing, sensual massages, or simply holding hands-on after-dinner walks.

We have included the detail of Dr Bartlik's advice as it captures the three most common issues and the three most common solutions that most couples interviewed for this book talked about. When a couple is sleeping separately purely because they need to sleep, there is usually a strong desire to ensure the physicality of the relationship is not lost.

Most nights (and I do mean most) I will go to Simon room after he has gone to bed and have a chat, lie on the bed with him and at a minimum, give him a kiss and a cuddle before he goes to sleep. We sleep with our bedroom doors open, so when we are both in our beds, and one of us is turning off the light to go to sleep, that person will call out and expect (and receive) a response. When Simon is dressed in the morning, he comes through and wakes me with a morning kiss and often on the weekend, one of us will wake and go through to the other's bed for a snoozy cuddle. We seek cuddles and kisses from each other often, and our sex life is healthy and not confined to the bedroom. Would we be having more sex if we slept together? We'll never know, but neither of us feels that we are missing out. We did make the effort to talk about how we would maintain physicality and intimacy when we decided to move to separate rooms, and from time to time, we will

remind each other if we feel one of us is backsliding
on our deal.
Sophia 52, married 13 years

Maintaining intimacy is an area where couples we interviewed spoke enthusiastically about 'keeping romance alive', and we can honestly say that no-one saw sleeping separately as a reason for less sex. Busy lives, children, stress and getting older were all cited as reasons for a reduction in cuddling, kissing and sex, but as noted in the last chapter, most interviewees felt the intimate part of their relationship benefited from being more rested. Stephanie Coontz,[120] director of public education for the Council of Contemporary Families in Chicago, said many couples are 'confident enough that they have a nice marriage, but they don't particularly like sleeping in the same room. I don't think it says anything about their sex lives.'

I have had two long-term relationships in which I
slept separately. For me, not sleeping together in
these relationships was a mature, pragmatic solution
to a problem and had no bearing on the strength, or
otherwise, of either relationship. As long as love and
intimacy were preserved then sleeping separately
was not a threat to the stability of the relationship.
In both relationships, the decision was not based
in anger, e.g., "I can't take this any longer, go to
the back/guest/spare room". We simply had our
own bedroom, decorated the way we wanted, with
the bed that we wanted, etc. The way we made
sleeping apart work was simply that was that was all
it was—sleeping apart. Sleeping separately meant

that we did not, at least in this aspect of our life
together, have the "considerable struggle, effort,
negotiation, inventiveness, tolerance, and perhaps
compromise" to be together. We slept separately, so
we slept better, felt better and happier and thus one
potential source of conflict/source of resentment and
anger was removed from the relationship, as long
as the non-sleep bits of the relationship, i.e. the 16
hours of the day when you are awake rather than
the 8 hours when you are asleep, were good then it
did not matter where we slept. I was perhaps lucky
that my partners understood the problem and were
willing to accept the solution of sleeping apart (I, of
course, realise that I could be accused of being guilty
of presenting just my 'happy' version of events to
support my arguments and that my partners may give
an entirely different account of the situation).
Neil, Sleep Expert, 55 years old

Couples do speak of a need to be more explicit about their actions and behaviour to ensure the full spectrum of intimate behaviours in their relationship are kept alive, but again, the most common tales told are of positive results.

There are two parts to plan for – maintaining the intimacy and maintaining the sex. I think the best way to give examples of what can be done is to hear from the couples who have already worked it out.

Maintaining the intimacy

For us, we are naturally close to each other and
maintain this by really strong communication. It's

a fundamental connection for us. We would feel
more distant when we haven't had the opportunity
to check in with each other each day. That's more
important than a good night or good morning
kiss. Not that they don't happen. We try to have
family dinners when we are home, which starts the
conversation, once the kids are in bed it's our time to
reconnect; 'download the day' with each other. We
might watch TV or just sit with a glass of wine and
swap stories. We are lucky that we work in the same
office so often drive to and from work together, and
that time adds to when we connect with each other.
We definitely don't feel that we are missing out on
any physical closeness by not spending every night
in bed together.
Neil, HR professional, 46, married 19 years

When I go to bed, I want to sleep. But if I go to bed
early enough, my husband will come and tuck me
in, we sit for 20 mins, and we chat and snuggle. If I
wake up early, like 5 am, I will go and have a snuggle
with him on the couch. We cuddle during the day, or
when we're watching TV, I'll put my head on his lap.
Suzette, 40, administrative assistant, married 17 years

It's important that each night before we go to sleep,
we spend at least an hour in bed together before one
of us goes off to the spare room to sleep. Some of
the time will be doing something alone; the other half
will be doing something together, like watching part
of a movie or a TV show. Sometimes Maree will 'nag'
me to make sure this happens, but it's nice to be

forced to do it – I actually appreciate that she does insist on it because I think I would miss it otherwise. We also have a double shower that we use together each night. We love standing in there chatting, catching up on the day, discussing things we need to – it's one of our 'alone time' things that we really enjoy. It's downtime away from the kids and life.
John, 33, medical professional, married 3 years

Each night we sit and have a glass of warm milk together at the kitchen table and talk about the day before we go up to our beds. We head off to bed at the same time and get up at the same time. We do spend a bit of time together because we are a team and we rely on each other.
May and John, both 66, retired, married 40 years

On the weekend Doug comes into my room and we spend hours in the bed together and that's when we catch up on the week because we are so busy. Even though we will speak to each other about four times a day during the week, it's still good lying next to each other and chatting. We have human touch, but it's not overly romantic – that's just not us – but it happens and it's important. We laugh a lot together, and that's really important. I'll sometimes send a text message to Doug in his bed that I would like a cup of coffee. He makes it and comes into my room and hops into bed. It's great. Most times on the weekend we end up with everyone in the bed, me, Doug and the three children. We really do love it.
Penny, 40, mother, married 14 years

One of the things we found really important is snuggling in bed together in the morning, not necessarily for sex. That whole snuggling up, waking up, chatting in bed – that closeness of being together in the morning is really important. Particularly on holidays, we make an effort then to wander into the other one's room at 5 am to have that waking up time together. All this is time together. It's not about sleeping together. It's about being together when the sun's coming up in the morning, and you are having a natter together about the world.

Melissa, 47, executive, married 27 years

For me, it's about cuddling. It's clichéd and girly, but I don't care. My partner has realised that I need to cuddle, to have the physical contact we miss out on by not sleeping in the same bed anymore. I ask him for cuddles and sidle up to him on the couch. He knows now that sitting on the couch to watch TV = cuddles of some type. I think there's some link to a primal need for touch? I'm a tactile girl, so I seek to have that need met often. My partner tells me that he often hopes the cuddles will lead to more, and sometimes they do.

Justine, 32, town planner

Maintaining the sex

Sex? If you want it, it's still there. If you need it, it's still there. If you want closeness, you can ask. If I want 'company' I'll ask my husband to sleep with me,

and that's fine – but it doesn't have to happen every night thank goodness.
Dianne, 52, education professional, married 30 years

Having not slept together for ten years, we have perfected sex on the couch. Even though we recently went back to sleeping together when the children stayed in their beds for a while, the couch still got a good work out.
Michael and Liza, 41 and 39, married 10 years

Sleeping apart has had absolutely no impact on our sex life. Having children certainly has, but we've gone from having daily sex to weekly at a minimum. And the sex happens wherever and whenever.
Caroline, 30, photographer, married 7 years

While we are not the best at talking about it, our sex life hasn't suffered. Since we've been sleeping apart we've managed to have two children – so I think that means it's okay. I still shower in the ensuite of the main room so am often in there, and things just happen. I would say that in some capacity, whether we use words or not, we both know when the other would like to have sex. For us, it's mostly demonstrated through actions towards each other. Sometimes one or the other will go out of their way to appear when the other is going to bed and then spend time together in the bed. I guess you sometimes have to make an effort to make it happen. Our arrangement is working well for both of us. I think that even if we were in the same bed, the

*amount of sex would be the same because we have
such different sleeping patterns.*
Leanne, 41, HR executive, married 15 years

*Maintaining intimacy in any long term relationship is
difficult. Let's face it; the fizz definitely fizzles after a
while! Since spending more and more nights sleeping
separately, my husband and I too had to find our new
kind of normal; a normal that is unique to us. For
us, it all comes down to one word: 'effort'. And not
just making an effort once or twice or even a dozen
times, for us it is about doing what we can every
single day to keep that passion alive and keep it on
track.*

   *Like anything in life that is fabulous and worth
fighting for we made the decision to openly and
honestly discuss how our sleeping dynamics were
detrimentally affecting our intimate time. We realised
that like everything else in our lives, for example
getting fit and eating right or planning an amazing
holiday, we have to make an effort and put time
into actively thinking about our sex life. We have
to make time to put some music on and sit on the
lounge together with a glass of wine. I have to make
the effort to wear that sexy little nightie I know he
likes when he comes home. He has to make the
effort to leave me sweet, naughty notes. Or if he
really wants to surprise me, and this is going to
sound crazy I know, but for me to come home from
work to a house that is spic and span and all the
housework done is an amazing aphrodisiac. I have to
say that of everything he does for me; this is a real
turn on because it means he is giving me the gift*

of downtime and that means we have more time to relax together. This is priceless, and it doesn't cost a thing, just 'effort'.

We both need to do these things; not all the time but often enough to keep things exciting yet not so often things become routine, stale and boring again. I know all these things sound clichéd, but they are clichéd for a reason … because they work. At the end of the day, we've realised that regardless of what bed we are sleeping in if we want to keep our love life and our marriage alive for many years to come then it all comes down to the effort we put in.
Emily, 30, international flight attendant, married 4 years

As for sex, well there's certainly not that spontaneity any more, but with three children, there probably wouldn't be anyway. But after having no sleep and waking up resenting the other person, there's definitely not going to be any spontaneity anyway. We're more likely to have sex now because I don't actually hate Doug anymore for keeping me awake. We've got pregnant since we moved to separate rooms, so I can guarantee you we've done it at least once. I believe that women with children are much more approachable in the morning than in the evening because of being so exhausted by everything you have to do. I am so appreciative that I can fall into bed and not have my husband throw his hand on my boob. But I am equally appreciative when he slips into my bed after I have had a good night's sleep.
Penny, 40, mother of three, married 10 years

There has been no impact on our sex life at all. Whoever is keener just goes into the other's room. If you can't sleep and the other person is awake, then you can go in there. It's really about being respectful of the other person. We've always been happy with our sex life, we still are, but if one person wanted more, then they ask the other. No problems.
Richard, 48, IT engineer, married 20 years

We still have sex, early at night because I can't stay up late. We've done the dinner, the bath, put our son to bed and then we spend time together, watching TV or reading, or we'll just lie down and talk. We are still intimate and have sex quite a bit. It's mainly in my bed though, as I fall asleep so quickly.
Charlotte, 24, teacher, married 1 year

Our biggest problem is where not if. I might be exaggerating a bit, but we are getting a bit more adventurous, and it's become a bit of a game recently. I like sneaking into her bed in the mornings and waking her with a cuddle, more often than not, we end up having sex. But, we have started to look differently at various locations around the house. I can honestly say that it's been an unexpected bonus and I'm loving the fact that my wife is acting like we were when we started dating. I'm not sure how long this will last, but at this stage, I can't imagine not having sex with my wife – it would have to be that there was something really wrong between us, not because of our situation with beds.
Mike, 52, landscape gardener, married 23 years

Our marriage is not built on our sex life. There's
so much more to us and who we are as a couple.
There's still all the intimacy we want and need. Prior
to recent illness, we still had a very active sex life and
separate beds have had nothing to do at all with a
reduction in how often we have sex.
John and Margaret, 58 and 50, married 30 years

We hope these stories go some way to dispelling any myths or mistruths that sleeping separately means the end of the intimate side of a couple's relationship. Basically, if you are sleeping apart and not having sex, it's because you have decided not to – not because you are victims of circumstance. In most instances, factors other than where you lay your head at night are far more likely to relegate your sex life to the bottom of the list of 'things I do with my partner'. Honestly, there are just as many couples sharing beds who rarely talk, kiss or cuddle and have a terrible or non-existent sex life.

So, I guess most of the people opposed to separate
beds only have sex in bed at bed time? Now I guess
the rest of us get to feel sorry for you.
Mangonel, www.slate.com

We have to share a bed? Are you serious?

For waders and divers, another plan to be made is what to do if you both have to sleep in the same bed for one or more nights. This comes in to play if you visit friends or relatives and need to stay over, or the friends and relatives come to your place and need one of your rooms, or you go on holidays.

On a personal note, Jennifer and her husband try to arrange two rooms wherever they find themselves sleeping at night. They are fortunate that both their parent's houses can accommodate their needs, but it's not always the case for staying with friends or when they go on holidays. They have accepted that holidays can sometimes cost a little more if they want a two-bedroom unit. The argument then is who gets the bigger room – they take it in turns; very civil. However, when they stay in capital cities and want to be central, two rooms is often an expense they can't stretch to. This is also an issue when they travel overseas. The main solution is for Jennifer to wear earplugs. However, as noted in the beginning of the book, three nights is about her limit. There have been times where Jennifer has slept on couches if the accommodation permits, and she never underestimate the power of a few glasses of wine. As they are quite active during the day on holidays, and that certainly helps to wear her out. Sometimes though, Jennifer just doesn't get enough sleep, but she can live with that for a night or two, here and there. For Neil, bedpartner snoring is not the issue, it is the mechanics of sharing a bed that disturbs sleep, so if a hotel bed is not at least 6ft (180cm) wide then he is more comfortable sleeping on the floor than sharing a bed. He particularly remembers the disappointment of entering his room in a very famous, venerable, hotel in New York to be confronted with what must have been the smallest double bed in the USA and spending the 4 nights of a romantic weekend sleeping on the floor.

Most couples interviewed used similar tactics. A common solution for families is to split children (who seem to be able to sleep through just about anything) across two rooms, allowing the adults to split themselves across the rooms as well. Often noted is the ability to have an afternoon nap while on holidays, or recognition that not being at work means the need for an alert mind is not as imperative. However, some solutions are far more creative (although for some separate sleepers, holidays will never be what they once were).

> I have sleeping tablets, specifically for the times when we have to share a bed on holidays. I use them for no other purpose except getting some sleep when I have to share a bed with my husband. Love him to death, by the way.

Lulu, 42, legal professional, married 6 years

> On holidays, we try to split the sleeping across two rooms with one of the kids in a bed with each of us. If separate rooms are not an option, then I bring earplugs and industrial ear defenders from his workshop—the kind that someone uses when they are jackhammering. It probably seems hard to understand how I can sleep in them, but I position the pillow so that I can. I tested it with my snoring parents, and it worked beautifully. Recently on a camping trip, he knew he would keep everyone up in the cabin we had rented, so he slept outside in a tent.

Suzette, 40, administrative assistant, married 17 years

> Holidays – I dread them! Why? If I want to sleep, I

have to wear earplugs. Why should I have to do that?
I have three children, and I want to be able to hear if
they need me. We recently went to Noosa for a night
and thought we could surely spend one night in a
bed together. Turns out – no, we can't. At about 3 am
I'd had enough of the snoring (which of course he
denied), so we had an argument, and he ended up
sleeping on the couch under one of my shirts.
Penny, 40, mother, married 14 years

Maintaining the plan

Once you have negotiated, refined, and implemented the plan, then you can sit back and relax – not. As social ecologist Peter Drucker says, "Plans are only good intentions unless they immediately degenerate into hard work." Many aspects of your relationship change as years pass and circumstances change. Relationships are not static; they constantly evolve, so don't become complacent.

When you have a plan in place, whether it's version 1, 2, 2a or version 35, take the time to regularly check-in with your partner to monitor how successfully the new arrangements are working for both of you. You may have a wide grin on your face and look years younger because of nights of uninterrupted sleep, but also take a genuine interest in how they are feeling about the new regime.

Revisiting the key reasons of why you wanted to sleep separately and letting your partner know how it's working is an important part of the whole process – kind of like making sure your golf swing goes all the way round to the back of your body and doesn't stop halfway just because you've hit the ball. Talking to your partner about any concerns that have developed, or indeed finding out if there are any positives they have discovered, will help to ensure the decisions made are sensible and potentially long-lasting.

Dr Timothy Sharp recommends that "With any planning or goal setting one of the most important things to do is constantly review what has been agreed. Making the plan is not the end of it – a couple should regularly reconvene and review the plan. If there are warning signs or indications that it isn't working then they need to constantly evaluate, review and make changes so that it is working."

> *When we finally decided to sleep apart, the first arrangement was Sunday–Thursday, so I could be rested for work. But after the first five to six months, I was beginning to dread Fridays because that was the night I would have to share with him. As much as I knew he would be upset, I just had to tell him that I couldn't do it. I had become used to having uninterrupted sleep so I figured why should I be exhausted on the weekends – that was my time to relax and do stuff, not spend Saturday and Sunday afternoons asleep to catch up. Loving someone does mean accepting them. I think my boyfriend has certainly had to learn that.*
> Justine, 32, town planner

Prioritising communication about your sleeping arrangements will ensure that you keep connected with your partner through combined monitoring of the situation and sharing of how the change has affected you both. Keeping the communication flowing will also allow you to do any necessary tweaking of the arrangements. This is likely new territory for both of you, and there is a strong chance you may not get it totally right, to begin with, so you need to keep your minds and mouths open to work out the finer details and leave you both confident in your choices.

This tweaking might involve reminding your partner that they need to pop in and share a cuddle with you before you go to sleep, or you both agreed that for half an hour every night, you will turn the television off and just chat. Some fine-tuning of agreed behaviours might also be needed. For example, 'I know we said we would try and have a cuddle every night, but with all our activities during the week, meeting this commitment isn't working. If we can promise to do it on the weekends, is that going to be okay?'

Once you are sleeping according to the new rules, make sure that any boundaries and behaviours that were part of the deal are honoured by both of you. They can always be re-negotiated if they are not working, but if you let them slip, you'll never really know if they were the right boundaries in the first place.

For example, the ritual of Jennifer's morning kiss from her husband. The reason she wanted (and still do) a kiss in the morning was because she didn't want Fraser to get up and go to work without her being aware that he had left the house. Her boundary there was about not missing out on the daily connections of life. There were a couple of times early in the arrangements that Fraser said he didn't want to wake her to give her the kiss, but for her, the kiss is more important than being woken – so he kisses her every morning.

If you don't talk to your partner about how the plans are working, necessary changes might not happen, and great successes may go uncelebrated; that would be a shame. Maybe you could arrange a conversation of this type with when you are having a cuddle on the couch, or one of you is visiting the other's room for some time together before you go to sleep?

> *There are times when we don't actually see or talk to each other for a few days because of my shifts and the fact that I'm downstairs and he's upstairs and we probably only eat together once a week. But John knows every move I make, my rosters, where I am, and I know where he is and what's happening in his life. Also, no major family decision would ever be made without a discussion between us taking place. This might mean that John comes to work to see me, we make the time for a phone call, or he comes early to catch me as none of these decisions are made independently. We respect each other too much.*
> Margaret, 50, retail manager, married 30 years

The bonus round

While there is a risk that the relationship might wobble a little when you move to separate rooms, there is also an equal possibility that one or both of you will find unexpected benefits when you experience single slumbering. All couples speak of the joy of having more sleep, but there's more to a bedroom than the sleeping.

> *I wake up earlier than Penny, so I have found that what I really enjoy is the whole thing of making a coffee, taking it back to bed where I read a magazine or surf the web. That, to me, is the one thing I like and that I would really miss if I had to share a bed again. Sometimes I do it for about two hours while everyone else is asleep. I'm in bed, I'm warm, and snug and I really enjoy it.*
> Doug, 43, IT project manager, married 14 years

> *Since I have the top floor of the house to myself now, I can have my bookcase in the lounge room with all my books in it, and all the sauce bottles and paper work for the business out in the kitchen. I always had to put those away. It's my den, and it's become important to me.*
> John, 58, building contractor, married 30 years

> *Having never thought I would sleep in a separate room to my wife, I am surprised by how well it works for both of us. One thing I love is if I wake up at 3 am, I just reach over, get my iPad. It's great.*
> Richard, 46, sports professional, married 21 years

> *My room is so tidy now, and I have decorated the room in a more 'girly' way – I wasn't allowed to before. I feel like I was trapped for so long, it's like owning something for the first time, owning my own space – this is mine. I can decorate it how I want, be*

in it how I want. No water bottles, no watches, no eating in bed, no chocolate. I have flowers next to the bed and some crystals and all new sheets and pillows. I find the experience liberating.

Anne, 44, senior manager, married 20 years

Since Sophie moved to the other room, I actually don't mind. I had always thought we would be sleeping together because it's the traditional thing to do, but this arrangement is actually working well for us both. I sleep when I sleep, I can get up and get a drink of water, go to the toilet … I can do what I want. I'm probably sleeping a fair bit better because it's less disturbed sleep. I'm passively enjoying it. I get up at strange hours, so it's convenient for me. I can get up early and then come back to bed again, and it doesn't disturb either of us. It's great.

Anthony, 62, education professional, married 25 years

What happens when the plan isn't working?

As Thomas Edison, supposedly, said: "*I have not failed. I've just found 10,000 ways that won't work.*"[121]

This chapter focuses unashamedly on solutions and success. However, we all know that plans can fail. In your path to separate sleeping nirvana, you are likely to encounter some bumps along the way. Some people might find mountains, and some may never solve their sleeping issues. Not every story has a happy ending. If you aren't finding your happy ending, you may need to look further than this book, as the issues are possibly bigger than where you lay your head at night. Sometimes just speaking to your GP is a good place to start.

When you are planning, though, include some thinking and talking about what might go wrong. Any good contract lawyer would support us in this advice. If you can foresee and prepare for pitfalls, the disappointment and frustration when they happen will be lessened.

The foreseen problems will range in scale, which will have an impact on how easily they can be solved. For example, smaller issues might arise, such as:

- When one of you wants to come into the other's bed, but the other doesn't want them in there.
- When neither of you wants to volunteer to move to the spare room.
- If neither of you wants to give up your room when you have so many guests that a surrender of one of your beds is required.
- If one of you feels they got a raw deal by not having access to cupboards or ensuite.
- If the person in the main room feels as though they are still being disturbed by the other coming into the room to get clothes, have a shower etc.

While smaller issues can have simple solutions, there may be some problems that are harder to resolve or situations where one of you is happy with the changes, but the other one isn't. How would you deal with the situation when one of you:

- doesn't like sleeping apart
- feels that you are growing apart

- is unhappy about changes to your sex life and the romance and physical aspects of the relationship
- feels that the arrangements agreed upon aren't working anymore
- can't deal with questions about the new arrangements?

These tough problems may not have quick, easy resolutions. They may require some external advice, but continuing to support, communicate and be open and honest with each other will certainly help as you work your way through these issues.

Pause for thought...

- Is your relationship in a place and space to be making plans to sleep separately?
- Does where you live offer some options to accommodate sleeping separately?
- How well do you and your partner plan for upcoming events? And more importantly, how well do you cope and deal with each other, and the situation, if a plan doesn't work?
- Do you know already if you are heading for the paddling or wading pool, or are you limbering up for an elegant dive into the deep end? And does your partner know about your plans? If not, how is he going to find out?
- How do you and your partner define intimacy? Is this something you can talk to them about if you were to sleep separately?

- Are you able to accommodate all the logistics of the plans you are making for your changed sleeping arrangements?
- Is there a trusted friend or family member that could help you come up with some creative suggestions to your particular sleep plan if you are stuck when thinking of solutions? How could you approach this person if you needed to?

SEVEN

What will the neighbours think?

'It is grossly selfish to require of one's neighbour that he should think in the same way and hold the same opinions. Why should he? If he can think, he will probably think differently. If he cannot think, it is monstrous to require thought of any kind.'

Oscar Wilde[122]

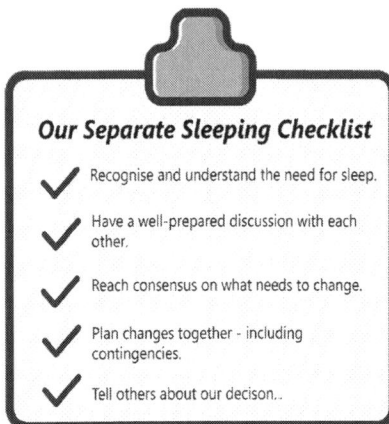

Our Separate Sleeping Checklist

✓ Recognise and understand the need for sleep.

✓ Have a well-prepared discussion with each other.

✓ Reach consensus on what needs to change.

✓ Plan changes together - including contingencies.

✓ Tell others about our decison..

When you have made the decision to sleep separately there will come a time when you may want to tell people what's happened. Or there may come a time when you are put in a position where the new arrangements are uncovered and you either choose to spill the beans about who is sleeping in which bed at your house, or are left in a situation where you have little choice but to do so. As with many other aspects of sleeping separately the sharing experience will be different for everyone. For some, telling others of your decision may cause as much disruption to your life as swatting away a fly, but for others letting people know of the new arrangements is more difficult than making the decision itself. Why? It's all tangled up in our version of what makes a successful life and wanting other people to think we're successful too.

A fundamental feature of humans is we want to be liked. Some of us are satisfied knowing there is just one person in the world who enjoys our company, whereas others require an entourage to pander them 24/7. Maslow's ubiquitous triangle of needs[123] has been telling us for decades that once we have all the basics in place (of which sleep is found on the foundation layer we might add), then we work to meet a range of other needs further up the pyramid. At the pointy end of the triangle are self-esteem, confidence, and respect from others, which are all gained through positive interactions with people that like us.

Seeking approval from others helps us meet Maslow's higher-order needs by making us feel good about ourselves, proud of our achievements, relevant to others' lives and valued by the people we care about – and there's no harm in admitting that. To have our needs met, we tend to behave in ways that we hope will continue to make us an attractive proposition. We work hard for our boss; we follow our parents' rules, we give our friends presents for their birthdays and engage in all sorts of social behaviours to oil the wheels of happy relationships and keep the ones we're out to impress coming back for more.

On a very basic level, we form two types of relationships in our lives. There are the ones over which we have little or no control – family, co-workers, neighbours. Then there are the ones we manage ourselves – friends and intimate partners. While we don't intend to go into the complexities of the interpersonal dynamics of all types of relationships, it is sufficient to say that when we seek approval (in whatever form) from any person, our behaviour is influenced to obtain that approval. What we say and do, how we act, our opinions shared and unspoken and our appearance, whether in clothes or deeds, are open to influence when we want someone to tell us that we are okay.

Some argue that being validated through others' approval is one of the strongest motivating forces known to man. However, on a day-to-day basis just knowing that there are people who like you and seek you out for a chat or a hug and can provide you with the necessary emotional and physical nourishment needed to encourage you to hop out of bed each morning.

Social approval is just as important. Psychologists describe social approval as a need, not a desire, and a psychological reality for healthy self-esteem. As social beings, our need to belong to a group starts young and stays forever. Again, it's an issue that's danced around many wise brains and filled many university libraries, so not one we're going to delve into too deeply here. But it does have an influence on the topic of this book. As has been noted, sleeping is a social behaviour that attracts social scrutiny. As a result, people around us feel that they can comment on our sleeping practices and therefore give us the 'stamp of approval, or the sigh of dismay', depending on what your bedroom behaviours are and what they think of them.

> *Our friends were interested to see that we had separate rooms and thought 'Well, this marriage is on its way out'.*
> Von, 72, married 55 years

A contributing factor to how much value you place on the approval of others is their relative importance in your life. The more important people are to you, the more value you place on the relationship and the greater their approval matters, or, better put, the more their disapproval matters.

So, when you and your partner are with other people and say, 'Hey, X and I have decided to move into separate rooms', how will the people in your life react? Will their reaction influence your behaviour and how you feel about the decision you've made?

Oh, the stigma of it all!

Let's get right down to it! The most common reason that separate sleeping is maligned is the stigma that says if you're sleeping separately, your relationship is in trouble – people speculate about the cause, from issues with your sex life to the end of the relationship. And there's no real surprise in that conclusion. A common response when two people engage in conflict is to avoid each other, so the judgement does have a sound anthropological basis.

An aunt who is 15 years older than me passed a comment on my husband and I sleeping in separate rooms – 'If we slept in separate beds that would be the end of our relationship'. I did worry about what she had said for a while, but I couldn't draw a comparison to my relationship and our situation. My uncle doesn't snore, which is a big difference.
Leanne, 41, HR executive, married 15 years

However, as with all generalisations, we are subjected to and subject others to, there are exceptions. So why can't we make the decision to sleep separately, then say to all those judgers and detractors, 'Don't worry, everything's okay' and just get on with it?

Well, lots of people do, and their friends and family are convinced over time that everything is indeed okay, and they aren't facing the support tasks that come along with the end of an intimate relationship. This was certainly Jennifer's situation, and nearly twenty years on, she thinks she has convinced everyone that Fraser and her are okay, which is a relief.

However, the social groupings some people find themselves in may not accept a simple statement of 'everything's okay'. Stop and think about some really strong opinions you have. What are they? For Jennifer, she is quite firm in the belief that every person has the right to a good night's sleep, as evidenced by what you are reading.

Most people have an opinion about what constitutes a 'good marriage' or a 'good relationship'. The notion of pairing with another in a committed relationship brings the expectation that you will spend a lot of time together, and be each other's social partner of choice, operating as a unit in life. It's not an unrealistic model given the cultural and social messages in the media and society. When this typical model is not adhered to, eyebrows begin to rise and murmurs of 'What's wrong?' start.

Some people I tell find it so confronting. When people hear we have separate rooms, immediately you see their faces drop and think 'Oh, there's something wrong with the marriage, why haven't you told me?' Women have taken me aside and asked if everything is okay. I didn't even think it would be an issue for other people, but I would see the shock on their faces.
Penny, 40, mother of 3, married 10 years

I don't know if I would tell anyone because I wouldn't want them to think there was something wrong with us. I don't want them to jump to the wrong conclusions – that there is something wrong, because there isn't.
Sophie, 60, retired, married 25 years

Recently I mentioned to a friend that my husband and I sleep separately. 'Oh, are you okay?' was her immediate reaction. I said we were fine and mentioned we were building another bedroom and she totally assumed that we were having marital

*problems. I told her that there were absolutely no
problems and that it was more about the fact that
I don't want to kill my husband because I am sleep
deprived.*
Suzette, 40, administrative assistant, married 17 years

*I don't promote or advertise it at all as people will
think there are cracks and vulnerabilities in the
relationship – it's nobody else's business, and I don't
want people to judge us on that. If it comes up, it's
not a secret, but I find it very persal.*
Amelia, 41, mother of two, married 12 years

*I don't necessarily care if people know. I don't go
out of my way to tell people, but don't deny it. I
don't have a problem talking about it. I think people
who react negatively to it are very old fashioned. It's
nothing to be ashamed of at all – it's just practical.
When my parents did it, it just made sense.*
Maree and John, 30 and 33, health professionals, married 3
years

*I'm very open about our situation, so get some
interesting reactions. People say 'It's not a real
marriage', but I tell them 'Different strokes for
different folks, and it's what works for us'.*
Caroline, 30, photographer, married 7 years

*Someone once told me I would never get married
because of my opinions about things like this,
and that is fine, actually. However, I do not think
you should let society decide on your sleeping*

arrangements because you are not married to them.
With the high divorce rate triggered over silly things,
why not do whatever it takes to make your marriage
better for you. If that means separate beds or
bedrooms, then go for it. Do what works for you and
not what is sanctioned by your neighbours.
Sweetbearies, www.slate.com

A 2007 article from the *New York Times*[124] considered the
point of view of builders and architects who were engaged
by people building and renovating to accommodate their
separate sleeping needs. Even these people recognised
the issues faced by people when it came to sharing their
decision.

Many architects and designers say their clients
believe there is still a stigma to sleeping separately.
Some developers say it is a delicate issue and call
the other bedroom a 'flex suite' for when the in-
laws visit or the children co me home from college.
Charles Brandt, an interior designer in St. Louis
said, 'The builder knows, the architect knows, the
cabinet maker knows, but it's not something they
like to advertise because right away people will think
something is wrong with the marriage'.

So many images in Western culture depict a good
relationship by showing a happy couple jumping into a
bed together every night. So, it's really no surprise that
so many people take their cues of what to do to be a
good couple from these images and are challenged by a
different model. When faced with a different way of doing

life well, some people become fearful. The unknown is a scary place, and some of us don't want our happy, successful life model tested by others. Because what if my model fails? Better the devil you know than the devil you don't!

For some, the sting of the stigma is closer to home and comes from themselves. Messages throughout their lives have told them that a couple should sleep together, and they may have judged others in the past on unconventional decisions that didn't fit with their own model. So, when faced with the situation where they are the ones not living up to their ideals of a good relationship, the internal conflict can send them into shame and guilt, making sure that any sleeping arrangements outside the norm remain secret.

> I would fret about it and think that I was a bad wife because the only time my parents ever slept apart was when they were having a fight and my mother locked my father out of the room. I have been brought up to believe that in a family, parents do everything together, they sleep together, they get up and make the bed together – that's what a good couple do. I don't think I will ever tell my parents that I am sleeping apart from my husband. I have only told one person at work that my husband and I have moved to separate rooms. There's a stigma that says there's something wrong that we aren't sleeping together, and I don't think I'll ever be comfortable about being in separate rooms. However, I do find the experience liberating.
>
> Anne, 44, senior manager, married 20 years

Realistically, the best way to chip away at the stigma that your relationship is in its death throes because you aren't sleeping in the same bed is with ongoing successful separate sleeping. The longer you sleep apart and stay together, the quieter the naysayers become. (And maybe give them a copy of this book)

What about my BFFs?

When we are young, our friendship groups happen to us, not by us. Friends appear in our life because of who we sit next to in class, who our mum makes friends with at the school gate or tuckshop, and who we live next door to. As we grow older, friendships are made more independently, through shared values, social norms, and social behaviours.

There is a wealth of psychology behind why we make friends with one person rather than another – but it's basically because they are like us, and they get us. They understand our sense of humour, our social decisions, and they like the things we like. Often there are characteristics we see in our friends that we would like for ourselves and that also attract us to them. Essentially, you share a certain amount of social assets with this person, so you hang out. Friends validate each other. That's why you seek them out over others because you are always approving of each other and have a lot of fun together.

Sometimes we make friends for aspirational reasons. We may seek out people in a different demographic to ourselves because they represent the type of person we want to be, or we are presented with an opportunity to mix with a group of people who are different to us, and suddenly, we have a different set of norms to learn about and demonstrate if we want to remain in the gang. These types of friendships may not have the foundations that allow for a level of honesty that you might have with other friends, but there is something in the social pairing you want, and one of those things is their approval.

Friends have their opinions too, and sometimes we find ourselves on the outer edge of a group because we aren't modelling the requisite behaviour to belong. We aren't wearing the right brand of clothes, being seen at the right restaurants or parties, drinking at the right bars or hotels, supporting the right football code (or even knowing what codes there are and that we are supposed to support a team) – or we aren't sleeping in the same bed as our partner.

There are people who like to present a façade of blissful happiness in their domestic life. For some, it's a very shiny badge of honour. What is a blissful domestic life though? There's the one often portrayed in the media of mum and dad being terribly good at whatever domestic arrangement works for them – both working or mum at home with dad as the breadwinner – the kids are happy and healthy, everyone gets on with each other, a fluffy dog plays enthusiastically in the back yard, and everyone has an untroubled life. (Just to confirm – mum and dad do sleep in the same bed every night, very happily, with lots of pillows and a great matching quilt and sheet set and coordinated, stylish nightwear.)

If this is your family and you are happy, then great! There is nothing wrong with this story, but it's just not everyone's story, and there would be a lot of people who don't want that story either. What's blissful to one is not blissful to another, and neither state of bliss is better than the other. The different definitions of blissful are what enables frameworks for judgement and disapproval. If you have friends, who either through actions or words, make it very clear they would never sleep separately to their partner, then it might be difficult to admit that you do – if you fear that they will disapprove of your decision. It's even tougher if you think that their disapproval might lead them to judge you negatively and not maintain your friendship anymore.

> *We don't tell a lot of people that we sleep in separate rooms. We had to put a system in place because sleeping together wasn't working. My room still looks like a spare room anyway, so no-one would notice the difference.*
> May, 66, retired, married 40 years

> *I've told my two best friends, and that's it. I don't need to be judged, and I know I have friends who will do that. When I'm with friends, and they are joking and laughing about their husbands snoring and keeping them awake at night, I join in. I have years of experience to keep telling stories. What would happen if they found out? I'll cross that bridge when I come to it, but I do think about that happening from time to time.*
> Maddie, 35, health professional, married 6 years

We don't like to think of ourselves as failures. And keeping friendships is a task at which we can fail. Sometimes our friends, their reactions to what we do and their opinions about us act as a social mirror. So, when you normalise your behaviour against people you consider your friends, but who have a different normal to you, you may not feel comfortable looking in that mirror. When it comes to sharing that you can't sleep with your partner anymore, you need to decide if sharing the information and risking disapproval is the right thing for you, or if you prefer to keep that type of information to yourself. Dr Timothy Sharp says that in most circumstances, most people outside a relationship don't know the ins and outs of how it works, and they don't need to. As in many other areas of your life, how important is it what other people think of you? It's a balancing act, but what's important to you and your partner should be the main priority to focus on.

My husband was out with his mates and telling them a story about how our son prefers my pink sheets to his blue sheets. When they found out the sheets were different colours because we have separate rooms they thought it was the weirdest thing ever and couldn't believe that we sleep in separate beds. In fact, lots of our friends question it or are really shocked and surprised by it. They think it's the strangest thing they have ever heard.
Charlotte, 24, teacher, married 1 year

Like any man, I, of course like the idea of going to bed next to and waking up next to my wife every day. This is what I have always equated to normal. It makes me sad when I wake up in the morning,

*and she is gone. It makes me frustrated when she
wakes me up in the night and asks me to leave. I
understand that sleeping together many nights is
just near on impossible for her with my restlessness
and snoring, and she reaches a breaking point. I
understand; but it still upsets me. We've had many
conversations together about how we need to create
a new kind of 'normal' that works for us. But I have
to be honest; I would definitely feel embarrassed
telling my mates that my wife and I don't share a bed
most nights. It's the ridicule and them asking 'What's
wrong with you mate?' that is still hard to face.*
Harold, 33, business development manager, married 2 years

Who you do and don't tell is an individual decision. You
will know which of your friends will cope and which ones
will feel challenged. Consider, however, that there may
be friends who although presenting a façade of a happy
home with perfectly sleeping babies and super happy
husbands snoozing the nights away next to them, maybe
thrilled to hear there are options available for them to
get a good night's sleep. They might be grateful that
someone has the courage, to be honest about the issue
and follow your lead.

There may also be people who are grateful to have
the opportunity to discuss the idea of separate sleeping
with you. It gives them the opportunity to find out how it
can work and how it might affect a relationship, positively
or otherwise.

*Even though we have had problems sharing a bed
for a while now, I really hadn't thought about moving*

to separate rooms until I spoke to a friend and found out he was doing it. I guess I just didn't think it was an option. I started telling my wife about what my friend did, and after a few conversations, we thought I should move to the spare room downstairs. I love it; my wife loves it. It's great. We've got a friend coming to stay for a few weeks soon, and I have to move back to the main room for that time. I'm not looking forward to having to give up my room.

Richard, 46, sports professional, married 21 years

I have had lots of interesting things said to me as I am very open about it. Some people are shocked, some people have said they wished they had separate rooms and others have then gone out and done the same thing.

Melissa, 47, executive, married 27 years

Often when I'm with friends, we will get on to the topic of snoring, and it often leads to 'Where do you sleep at night'. Sometimes the question comes up 'Does your wife put up with it?' Some say 'Yes', and some say 'No, I have to sleep in another room.' It's as simple as that. We're all in the same boat. I feel good to know there are others in the same situation as me. None of my friends say they are in another room for any other reason, so I don't know of any other. We talk seriously about it. If there are other people around it can be a bit light-hearted, but one-on-one the conversations can get serious. Some wished that they didn't have to be out of their own rooms, some miss their wives. No-one's embarrassed; they

are more concerned about whether it's impacted on
their intimacy. In some cases it has, and they want
to talk about it. What they are looking for is – it is the
same for you? Is everything alright? And they are not
as intimate – but for them, there are probably other
factors that impact on the fact their intimacy is not as
they want it. It's definitely more than just sleeping in
separate rooms. I've probably spoken to about three
close friends about it, and we do agree that we don't
like keeping our wives awake but don't have issues
with sex.
Matt, 47, senior manager, married 20 years

Those close to you may not be the only people with whom you choose to share your separate sleeping news. While most people don't go out of their way to constantly announce their night-time domestic arrangements, there may be times where the topic is raised or an opening for a discussion on the issue presents itself and before you know it, you're sharing your personal story with someone you've just met. As veterans of this practice, we have some advice on the array of responses that you might be presented with as well as how to deal with them if you do choose the virtuous path of truth as a separate sleeper.

You do what?

While Jennifer never starts a conversation with, 'Hi, I'm Jennifer, and I sleep in a separate room to my husband,' she certainly doesn't shy away from talking about this aspect of her life. Often in conversation, she will mention 'my husband's bedroom' or 'my bedroom', or the context of the conversation is such that the topic is appropriate to broach. Neil takes the same approach.

Having a particular interest in all things sleep and sleeping arrangements, we both enjoy hearing other people's view on the practice and enjoy hearing their stories as separate sleepers or dedicated co-sleepers themselves. We are interested to hear anecdotes about how the range of sleeping misdemeanours is managed by couples. There is also a cheeky side of Jennifer that enjoys challenging social norms, so she brings an enthusiastic interest to the debate of 'one bed or two'. Neil often deals with the topic in a more formal way.

These are the most common responses we have encountered. You may recognise some of these – and be able to add some more types to the list.

The Head Tilter

As this person listens to you explain that you sleep separately to your partner, their head starts to tilt – not too much, to either the left or the right. You are left thinking – is there something wrong with your neck? While there may indeed be a spine-related injury they're dealing with, the Centre for Non-verbal Studies says that a head tilt can be used to show friendliness or be one of several self-protective gestures.

Potentially, these people think your relationship is in such dire straits that you need more friends. Or maybe they are thinking, 'I wonder if my partner wants to sleep separately from me?' So, the head is tilted as a preemptive pose that will enable them to spring into action in case this is a reality. We are conjecturing, of course.

There is a tilt that we call the 'pity tilt' – you can see it in their eyes. Often the Tilter tries to encourage an admission from you that there must be just a little something wrong with the relationship for you to take such drastic steps. Both authors have had a couple of Tilters encourage them to admit to them that there is something wrong in our relationships. 'It's okay, you can tell me' has been offered as a safe haven for our confession. 'Don't you miss the cuddles all night?' they coo. 'Don't you want to snuggle next to your partner, fall asleep and wake up next to them in the morning?' The answers to these questions are 'yes' and 'yes', hastily followed by 'but what is more important to us is getting enough sleep to function, etc'.

How to respond to a Tilter: What we would love to do is reach over to the Tilter and straighten their head for them, but there are all sorts of issues such as social boundaries and good manners we would break if we did that. We know you can't change opinions in one conversation, so a suggested response to them (and it's going to be a repeated suggestion in the next couple of pages) is to assure the Tilter that all is well in your relationship, this is the solution that works well for you and your partner, and as individuals, we have the ability to make decisions that work best for us. You might also offer the Tilter some more information about sleeping separately – possibly throw in a few statistics – so they have a greater understanding of people who are in a happy relationship, but just can't sleep in the same bed at night. It's just logic, not the end of the world.

The Seat Shifter

Seat Shifters do not want to hear about your separate sleeping. There is something about the practice that unnerves them so that they start moving around in their seat and employ every non-verbal tactic available to let you know you have strayed into taboo territory with them. Most commonly, they will move from an open body position to a cross-legged one that has the leg closest to you crossed away from you. They will angle their body away from you as well. This can be uncomfortable if you are in a small group.

Next comes the gentle, polite, winding down of the conversation. They will stop talking as much and move to 'mmms' and nods as you continue to try to engage them in the conversation, they appeared to be quite happy having about three minutes ago.

Being mostly polite people, we respect these cues and finish the topic as seamlessly as we can, letting the Seat Shifter return to a happy space by moving the conversation on to the weather or a recent sporting event.

An educated guess tells us that this topic is off limits for them. Not wanting to exacerbate their uncomfortableness we have never pursued Seat Shifters to find out why they respond so. Whether it touches on a boundary of what constitutes their version of a good relationship, or crosses the line of what's appropriate to talk about in polite company, or is something they do but don't want to disclose … who knows?

How to respond to a Seat Shifter: We really do think the best thing to do is be as polite as you can and gently move away from the topic. If the Seat Shifter wants to talk about it again, they will – that has happened to both of us on rare occasions. Everyone's level of social comfort around personal topics is different, and it is important to respect that. Depending on where you are in the conversation, it could be worthwhile to drop in that your relationship is okay. This would help Seat Shifters to feel that they could get back to you if there was something they wanted to know or talk about further with you.

The Frowner

The Frowner is like the Tilter but has a more judgemental edge. Whereas the Tilter might be overcome with pity, want to take you home and cuddle you all night in bed, the Frowner is usually communicating that 'couples don't sleep separately'. A frown unarguably says disapproval, so the Frowner is sharing their disapproval and displeasure at what you are telling them. They don't feel uncomfortable; they feel self-righteous and confident that their opinion on the practice is correct. And guess what? You have it all wrong.

The Frowner is as confident about why you shouldn't sleep separately as you are about why you should, so this one could be a battle of wills if you want to engage them. We like engaging Frowners as all views and thoughts about couples sleeping together intrigue us. If you are feeling a bit provocative and up for a rowdy and robust discussion, the Frowner is a great sparring partner.

Be careful though, the Frowner might be a version of the Seat Shifter, and their disapproval is about raising such a personal topic when you don't know them all that well. You may have caught them off guard, and while their level of discomfort is not as pronounced as the Seat Shifter's, the frown might be enough of a cue for you to look outside and see what the clouds are up to.

How to respond to the Frowner: First, if you think the Frowner is disapproving of the practice of separate sleeping, you might want to gird your loins and take them on in a feisty debate, or depending on the context, back down and pull out that trusty weather conversation. Second, if the frown emanates because of the personal nature of the topic, or the time and place of the conversation, changing to an innocuous topic will allay their concern and hopefully have them using their best-smiling muscles within seconds.

The Secret Sharer

The Secret Sharer is one of our personal favourites. They often listen intently to the explanation of your sleeping arrangements because they too are separate sleepers but don't tell anyone. They question your motivations, how you made it happen, how your relationship is going now, but what they most want to know is how you go about telling other people. Do you tell other people? What do you say? What do the other people say? Are you embarrassed? What do your parents think? What do your friends think? What do the pets think? Where do the pets sleep? What do the kids think? Have you told your workmates? What did they say? How many people do you tell? Why? Depending on their enthusiasm, it can be hard to get a word in.

Because Secret Sharers are separate sleepers themselves – some in the wading pool, some in the deep end – they want to know how you manage the fact that other people know about your separate sleeping. They want to know this because they don't tell anyone about their separate sleeping. Whether they are looking for a roadmap for how to tell others, or they want to vicariously revel in the social freedom you enjoy, they just can't get enough of your war stories of disclosure.

The Secret Sharer will often take the opportunity to disclose to you that they too sleep separately. This will only happen in a one-on-one situation. If you start your story in a group of people, the Secret Sharer will wait until they can capture you alone to quietly say, 'My partner and I sleep separately too'. What you then have is a sharing of details and the opportunity to make someone's day and normalise their life. I always feel honoured when a Secret Sharer confides in me, but I must admit I do tend to keep them cornered too, to drill down into why they are reluctant to share their situation. Much like the Frowner, they have a story to tell, and I am always genuinely interested in hearing the story.

How to respond to the Secret Sharer: First and foremost – don't break their confidence. It's a privilege to have someone share such personal details with you and not one to be taken lightly. By explaining your thought processes about why it's okay to share your situation with others, you help the Secret Sharer see that there is a social acceptance of the practice that can be gained from assuring others that separate beds don't mean the end of the relationship. Without patronising the Secret Sharer, find a way to affirm their sharing. We have never taken on the role of separate sleeping evangelists, so are not inclined to free them from their shackles of shame and personally, we don't think after hearing their confession, that introducing them to others as, 'This is Pete. He's a teacher and a father of three and hasn't slept in the same bed as his wife for the last five years' is the right thing to do. We do advise affirming their choice and teaching him the 'separate sleeper secret sign' – just kidding. That hasn't been designed yet.

The I-want-to-hug-you

I-want-to-hug-you listens to your story with a look of immediate empathy and warmth. They may reach out and touch you on the arm, or put their hand to their mouth as they take little gasps at each revelation you share. When you have told enough of your story for them to realise how similar their story is to yours, they will disclose that they too are a separate sleeper. I-want-to-hug-you is more likely than the Secret Sharer to disclose there and then, irrespective of the company, that they are in the club.

I-want-to-hug-you is just so glad to hear that there are others out there that share their situation and they want to show you how much they appreciate the camaraderie by adding a physical element to the conversation – this is when the hug or the further arm touch might happen. You may actually be the first person that I-want-to-hug-you has come out to, so don't treat their sharing lightly. They are not as embarrassed about their choice as Secret Sharer, but being human, they appreciate the chance to normalise a behaviour they may previously have thought they were the only ones engaging in.

Similarly, I-want-to-hug-you might latch on to you and want to know more because they hadn't even thought that this option was available to them. In fact, if this is the case, they may cry when they hug you because a light in their otherwise darkened, sleep-deprived life has been turned on by your sharing. Depending on your own social boundaries, you have to decide how you manage a teary, but grateful stranger.

How to respond to I-want-to-hug-you: We all like to know we're not alone in the world, especially when we choose a path less travelled. We want to meet the other travellers on our narrow path. It's exciting when we do. Welcome, I-want-to-hug-you with as much enthusiasm as you are comfortable displaying. The SSC (Separate Sleepers Club) has a membership equivalent to only 25% of most Western cultures, so while an important group in society (because we're so well-rested and therefore highly functioning social contributors) we aren't the majority. I-want-to-hug-you might want to share the details of their story with you, so plan ahead for meeting this person and think about how much you want to share and hear.

The Overly-Interested Questioner

Overly-Interested Questioners wants to hear all the details about your separate sleeping arrangements for one of two reasons. Either they are thinking about doing it, or their partner has been talking about doing it. Overly-Interested Questioners are on a fact-finding mission, and you have presented yourself as a personal 'Separate Sleeping Wikipedia' page. They are not going to miss this chance to click every hyperlink in your brain. Once you identify the Overly-Interested Questioner, it's your chance to speak proudly and confidently about your arrangements. These people are great to engage in conversation because you have something they want, so you are in the driver's seat.

You may want to take your time as you meticulously outline your separate sleeping arrangements and how it's been a life-changing experience for you, or choose a Reader's Digest version to give them a taste of what life could be like for them. You may indeed choose to hand the driver's seat over to the Overly-Interested Questioner and let them probe your expert knowledge bank. Whatever method you choose, it might be a good idea to get comfortable.

How to respond to the Overly-Interested Questioner: Be ready with facts. Also, be ready to answer a lot of questions that might plumb un-thought of depths in terms of detail. Consider asking them questions yourself to help them clarify their lines of enquiry. Be patient with Overly-Interested Questioners – they may be developing the questions on the run, so won't always be precise and methodical in their approach. And I warn you again, find a comfortable spot: you might be there for a while.

The That's-Interesting-Tell-Me-More

These people are simply interested in hearing your story and your thoughts about separate sleeping. They don't judge; they just listen. That's-Interesting-Tell-Me-Mores may be separate sleepers or they may not. They are just folk who are keen to have a good chat about a sociological behaviour and hear what other people in the world are up to. No surprises, no twist in the tail. Enjoy!

Doin' it for the kids

How you treat the task of telling your children about mum and dad's sleeping arrangements depends on the age of your children. If you have been sleeping separately since your children were youngsters, then you may only have to explain the situation if they ask questions following a sleepover at a friend's place where 'My friend's parents do this really weird thing and sleep together'.

After taking questions from a friend about the stability of my relationship because my husband and I weren't sleeping in the same room, she then asked, 'How do the kids feel about it?' I explained that it happened when my older one was five or six years old, so the kids don't know any different.
Suzette, 40, administrative assistant, married 17 years

Our kids think it's completely normal. They might think that sharing a room with a partner is abnormal.
Melissa, 47, executive, married 27 years

However, any explanation to young ones will probably be the same, no matter whether you are letting them know of an impending move to separate rooms or are giving them a rationale for your decision. This is another one of those situations where you will know what is best for you and your children, so you are in complete control regarding the level of detail you share and the emotion you create in explaining the situation. Their age and understanding of the dynamics of a mummy/daddy relationship will obviously impact on these factors.

Much like the concern raised by adults, some children might look at mummy and daddy heading to a different room at night and wonder if it might be leading to different houses in the not-too-distant future – 'like it did for Billy and Belinda at school'. Obviously, the key information that children need is to know that mummy and daddy are okay. This is easily evidenced by ensuring there are lots of cuddles and kisses between you, and again, depending on their level of understanding, having a discussion with your children about the stability of a relationship not being affected by where you sleep at night.

> *I constructed a story of the King and Queen's chambers for our children. So, when they come into my bed in the morning on the weekends, they think it's fun to come into the Queen's bed. When the King then comes in too, they think it's even better. They see that mummy and daddy still love each other because we're all in mummy's bed together laughing. Sometimes they go into Doug's bed too for a chat in the mornings.*
> Penny, 40, mother of 3, married 10 years

At a minimum, don't leave children wondering why their mummy and daddy are different to their friends' mummies and daddies who sleep in the same bed each night. And discussing the issue also presents an opportunity to teach your children that not everyone is the same and that relationships can be successful in many different ways.

Another situation you may find yourself facing is the inquisitiveness of friends of your children during sleepovers at your house. While it isn't up to you to educate other people's kids about the birds and bees, you don't want your children to feel uncomfortable if their friends' question, what is to them a strange arrangement. Something as simple as 'We sleep in separate rooms because we keep each other awake' is all that is needed to allay concerns. You may also want to coach your children to provide a simple explanation to their friends if the need arises. You may also choose to say nothing unless questions are asked by children or their parents.

When our children had friends coming to stay over I would see them looking perplexed that their friend's mum and dad were going to separate rooms when they went to bed. I could see them trying to process 'so the mum's bedroom is upstairs and the dad's is downstairs'. I think my kids just explained that it was normal in our house and it didn't really seem to bother them.
Brooke, 52, educational professional, married 30 years

Be mindful of your own child's developmental stage, as we all remember the cringe-worthy things our parents said to our friends. It would be nice if you could avoid making your child a social pariah with an overly-detailed explanation of you and your partner's personal issues.

Be strong, stay strong and sleep well

The Greek philosopher Heraclitus is attributed the iconic quote that "The only constant in life is change". This is certainly the case with social behaviour. Humans don't stop evolving and how we socialise has always been and will always be an area of change and challenge. We have evolved from sleeping separately to snuggling in a small space together, but maybe that is not proving to be the solution for everyone anymore. Klösch[125] notes that 'Separate bedrooms are becoming less of a taboo topic for couples. Separate sleeping arrangements are being chosen more and more often by pairs, and not just because of snoring...the double bed and sleeping together as a pair are products of cultural and historical processes, not biological necessity.' He goes on to say 'The days are gone when sharing a bed was seen as an indication of the health of the relationship ... separate beds and bedrooms can be a clear and visible sign of a lively and dynamic relationship.'

> *I think a marriage is whatever two people decide it is. It's what they decide what works for them. But a lot of people are worried about what the impression is that they give to others for fear of what will be said. I do feel that my husband is uncomfortable with it being an open topic, so I wouldn't raise it to prevent him feeling awkward.*
> Kaye, 66, together 14 years

> *We only tell people if it comes up. A lot of friends and all our extended family know what we do and*

why we do it. I think our attitude and approach to the situation makes other people feel okay about what we are doing. They see our relationship is okay, so we think that puts them at ease. We sleep in separate rooms because it's convenient for us. That's what we tell people.

Richard and Catherine, 48 and 46, IT engineer and health professional, married 20 years

If you know that sleeping separately to your partner is the right choice for you and for your physical and mental health, then be confident in that decision. There is no compulsion to share the decision or the details if you don't want to. But know that the decision is the right one for you and don't feel as though you have to justify it – publicly or silently – because it's different from the norm.

If you are confident that the reason you and your partner sleeping separately is not to create a smokescreen for more prominent issues in your relationship, then that needs to be evident when you talk about what you are doing. If you feel you are sleeping separately because there are more significant issues in your relationship, then it's probably a good idea to get brave and deal with those issues.

Telling others is all in the delivery. Share it nervously, and it will be received that way. Share it calmly and assuredly, and while you may not invoke immediate acceptance and approval from those who doubt or disapprove, you will at least begin the conversation with them from a better starting point. Many times, words are ignored when they are overshadowed by the vibe we pick up from the person who is telling us something. How you feel about your separate sleeping will influence your 'vibe', so think about your non-verbal behaviours as well as the words you use when conversations on the topic pop up. Dr Timothy Sharp recommends 'Get comfortable with it yourself, explain your circumstances to those you want to as best you can, when and where you want, and for others, try to not worry it. The most important thing is you and your happiness and health and well-being within the relationship, and if other people don't get it, well sometimes they won't – you can't please all the people all the time.'

Sleeping separately, and being open about the fact that you do, is about confidence in your decision, confidence in the reasons for your separate beds, and confidence in yourself and your partner.

Pause for thought...

- How do you feel about telling others of your choice to sleep separately or have some type of alternative sleeping arrangement?
- Do you feel confident about your decision, and do you think this confidence will come through if you were to speak about your separate sleeping?
- Do you have, or do you need to develop strategies to cope with negative reactions from other people?
- How do you react when other people speak about their sleeping arrangements? Are you aware of how you react?

- What facts do you have prepared if you are not openly comfortable talking about your arrangements, but find yourself in a situation where you don't have a choice?

EIGHT

Night night, sleep tight

Towards the end of 2012 and close to finishing the first edition of this book, Jennifer went with a friend to see the movie, *Hope Springs*, expecting to have a bit of a light-hearted laugh at an unashamedly middle-aged girly flick. However, as the opening scene unfolded, her eyes rolled in her head with dismay. Meryl Streep's character readies herself in a bathroom and then appears in the bedroom of her husband, played by Tommy Lee Jones. Immediately we know it's HIS bedroom, not theirs. Her husband rebuffs her romantic overtures, and she retreats to her bedroom, licking her emotional wounds. Again, her bedroom is very obviously the main room that used to be theirs. The movie epitomised every cliché of what separate rooms can signify for a couple. It screamed, 'You are in separate rooms because your marriage has failed'.

Jennifer was tempted to jump up in the cinema and shout to everyone, 'It doesn't have to be this way. Sleeping in separate rooms does NOT mean your marriage is over', but she thought she would save her friend the embarrassment. For those who have not seen the movie, it traces the attempts of a couple in their fifties to reinvigorate their failing marriage. The film relies on every cliché about what can go wrong in a marriage between an older couple – lapsed communication, no sex life to speak of, ill-fitting and dull clothing, and an over-reliance on each other and television to fill their lives. It really epitomised for her everything that can go wrong in a relationship – if the couple chooses to let that happen. And the sad reality is that in 2023, this image is still being trotted out by the media – happily though, less so. It all depends on how enlightened your media sources are.

The reality is that every couple, whether dating or married, together for a short while or a lifetime, has the choice to make their relationship be what they want. Not what the movies, the television, their family, or their friends say it should be. This is the central message of this book.

You define your relationship, and you determine what is good for you and what isn't.

Sleeping apart does not mean your relationship is falling apart.

- Sleeping apart does not mean your relationship will fall apart.
- Sleeping apart from your partner does not define your relationship.

Sleeping in the same bed every night won't save a troubled relationship. We don't deny that sharing a bed is the cornerstone of some people's relationship and the glue that helps them stick together, but it is not everyone's glue.

We've said it before, and we'll say it again – relationships are tough. Every relationship is tough, and the closer we become to a person, the more likely that person is to see all the bad bits of us and vice versa, which is what creates the hard work. But we also know that good things come from hard work.

Much of the advice provided in this book could be used to approach a range of relationship issues. The core messages of the advice are; work hard to have strong, honest communication with your partner and respect each other. These are neither new nor revolutionary ideas, but the fundamental skills needed to make any relationship work. As Jennifer says about her own relationship:

As far as my relationship with my husband is concerned, I do know that we are missing out on something by not sharing a bed every night. But this is just the same as we are missing out on something because we don't get up and exercise together every morning, or have a dedicated date night with each other, or fervently support a football team together. However, there are lots of other 'somethings' that we have in our relationship that other couples don't have. Fraser and I simply cannot sleep together. Love each other dearly but can't sleep together. We're certainly not alone, and I'm definitely not worried about the fact that we don't sleep together because I've now met so many happy, healthy couples –

*some together for nearly 50 years – who don't need to sleep in the same bed every night to keep their relationship on track. So I know that we aren't alone or unusual in our decision to have separate rooms. And nearly 20 years into our relationship, I know it's been the best decision **for us**.*

All the couples we have interviewed were asked how sleeping separately had impacted on their relationship, and if given a chance, would they change their current arrangements. Most of them would like to be sleeping together but know they can't, so they are happy with their current arrangements. Others, however, don't wish to change their current arrangements because they enjoy the benefits of sleeping alone while knowing they have a successful and happy relationship.

I'm happy at where we're at now. We have flexibility to sleep together or apart and don't need a more formal arrangement.
Ann, married 19 years

Given a choice, we would keep the same arrangement – the way we have it now. We recently talked about moving the new baby into a room of her own, and I suggested Doug's room. Straight away he said 'no' and that we would build downstairs before that would happen.
Penny and Doug, married 14 years

It would be great to be able to sleep in the same bed every night, definitely. But we've decided that this

*arrangement is just better. I get a good night's sleep;
she gets a good night sleep. Everything's cool. We
still love each other. There's no problem.*
Matt, married 20 years

*The simple fact is we have a lot of sleep
incompatibilities, so we both like having the freedom
of our own beds and rooms. We're very happy to
have separate rooms, but we do both like that our
rooms are connected. It gives us a togetherness.*
Richard and Catherine, married 20 years

*We're happy with the current arrangements. We get
along better because there's no resentment because
we are sleeping better. Life works better when at
least one of us is well rested. I couldn't imagine life
with both of us sleep deprived.*
Suzette, married 17 years

It's just a different version of normal.
Brooke, married 30 years

*We're past thinking that we are missing out on
anything. You think when you get married or move
in with another person that they are going to be
the last person you see at night and the first one
in the morning. After realising there were some big
problems about all the bits in the middle, we got over
that rapidly. I'm happy with the current arrangement.
It's what's kept us together.*
Caroline, married 7 years

Having felt like I was trapped for so long, I feel like

I own something for the first time. I own my own space. This is mine. I can decorate it how I want and be in it how I want. Now that I see it can work, I don't think it's odd anymore. I think it will keep us sane.
Anne, married 20 years

I don't feel that we are missing out on anything. I think we are gaining a fresher outlook each day. I don't think I'm losing anything and as long as my husband is open and honest with me and lets me know he's not losing out on anything, then I will be happy.
Charlotte, married 1 year

We have an inseparable bond that isn't affected at all by sleeping in separate rooms. We're like two old oak trees planted next to other, and our branches are growing together entwined as we get old together.
John, married 30 years

The constant evolution of human relationships assures us that what was unthinkable twenty years ago is now not only thinkable but probably in practice in contemporary society. Our generation has seen divorce become socially acceptable; de facto relationships become as valid as marriage and same-sex relationships commonplace and mainstream. How and where a couple arranges to sleep should be afforded the social generosity given to other behaviours that push the boundaries of what a couple 'should do'.

We cannot know if sleeping separately speaks of issues that go beyond your need to have a good night of uninterrupted sleep. That is your personal domain. What we can tell you is that as part of a happy and healthy relationship, sleeping in a separate bed every night, or just some nights, means little. Done well, it should help a happy and healthy environment flourish because both people feel valued, heard, and respected. And they are getting great sleep to keep them functioning.

When you feel confident and comfortable about what you are doing, that infiltrates all that you say about it to others. You don't have to advertise your personal decisions, but nor should you feel embarrassed about making such a practical decision. It's just sleeping at night – no-one's going to lose an eye or a limb over the decision.

When Neil lectures he often jokingly says that the most effective way of improving your sleep is divorce, but hopefully we have shown you that there is no need to go to that extreme, sleeping separately while in a loving relationship is perfectly natural and absolutely nothing to be embarrassed or ashamed about. Sleep is a biological need and a fundamental human right.

- Why compromise your quality of life, your physical, mental, and emotional health and indeed your relationship for a recent social construct?
- Are the opinions of newspaper 'relationship experts' really more persuasive than the scientific literature?
- Is the fear of 'what people might say' keeping you from sleeping better?
- Can a pattern of sleep practised for only a few hundred years by a small, culturally distinct

population, really be considered as the normal'
way of sleeping?
- Why have we fallen for this unscientific nonsense,
are the negative effects on our health happiness
and relationships worth it?

In a nutshell, there is no good thing of which to speak
about poor sleep. Whatever disturbs your sleep should be
managed appropriately to reduce the disturbance, and for
many of us, that includes our partners.

So, we cannot stress the point enough...

IT IS PERFECTLY NATURAL AND NORMAL FOR ADULT HUMANS TO SLEEP SEPARATELY

(We do hope the bolding and the font size conveys our
stance on the topic.)

We also hope we have given you enough information,
questions to challenge your thinking, and practical advice
about how you can get a good night's sleep.

So go forth and sleep.

If you need to name your new way to sleep a 'sleep
divorce', then do so with confidence. But we do both
hope that after reading our book, you only sleep apart...
not fall apart.

Night, night.

APPENDIX 1

The science of sleeping together

In the years since Jennifer and I first started talking about separate sleeping, there have been many scientific publications relating to the subject; below we have summarised the recent scientific work for the sake of completion. The style of the following section is more scientific (or as Jennifer described it 'dense') and there is no need to read it, it merely presents additional evidence to what we have already said. However, if you do persevere, you will hopefully see there is nothing in the research that changes the central message of our book.

A 2014 estimate using nationally representative data from the National Social Life, Health, and Aging Project showed that nearly 80% of married older adults, in the USA, slept with their spouses.[126] So one might legitimately ask why do they do this, why do couple sleep together?

Couples sleep – Concordance

Pankhurst and Horne conducted the first study to objectively measure the influence of bed partners on sleep in 1994.[127] They found that men showed a significantly greater number of discrete movements during sleep than did women. Overall, 5-6% of all 30-second sleep epochs contained such movements, with about a third of these movements being common to both partners. This concordance was highest in younger couples. Female bed partners reported being disturbed more often by their partner than was the case for male partners. Subjects sleeping with a partner showed a greater number of discrete movements than matched subjects who slept alone. Movements decreased during the temporary absence of the usual bed partner. Couples seemed unaware of the similarity in the timing of their movements during sleep, and most reported sleeping better when their bed partner was present. These results show the disconnect between subjective feelings of good sleep and objective evidence.

Following Meadows et al.[128] a paper from 2005, Gunn, et al.[129], in 2017 also examined minute-by-minute concordance in couples' actigraphy-defined sleep-wake patterns but additionally investigated how attachment style and marital satisfaction relate to this concordance. They found that wives' ratings of marital satisfaction may be more closely connected to concordance than husbands' ratings.

Later, Chen 2018[130] demonstrated that there are substantial discordances in older couples' bedtimes and wake-up times. Differences in bedtimes were associated with an increase in the psychological distress score, and these patterns were more pronounced on the weekends. The study showed that only 15–25% of older couples slept or woke up within 20 min of one another. Having a different sleep schedule from one's spouse is in itself a stressor because it affects their capabilities to perform their usual and desired activities.[131] Adults who go to bed earlier than their spouses may be disrupted when their spouses turn the light on, watch TV, or engage in noisy activities as well as their sleep being disrupted by the activities of spouses who wake up earlier in the morning. Furthermore, stress from differences in sleep timing may increase over time[132] and can cause conflicts in marital relationships.[133]

Lee et al.[134] also investigated sleep covariation within couples and found that sleep duration covaried within couples on a daily basis, indicating that, within a couple's relationship, how long one partner sleeps at night has a proximal effect on how long the other partner sleeps that night.

More recently Walters et al.[135] reported the first examination of dyadic sleep and wake concordance (time spent in shared sleep/wake) and wake transmission (how frequently a person's wake bouts were immediately preceded by a wake bout in of their bedpartner's) within a sample of cohabiting couples where one member was seeking treatment for insomnia. They found that partners of individuals with insomnia receive more frequent wake transmissions than those with insomnia, indicating that having a bedpartner with insomnia is disruptive to sleep. Their findings indicate there are two potential bedpartner disruption processes occurring in insomnia. First, disruption from a partner could perpetuate or increase wake transmissions and thus insomnia symptoms for some individuals. Second, disruption caused by the patient with insomnia to their bedpartner leads to interrupted sleep for the otherwise healthy sleeping partner, although the disruption to a bedpartner caused by someone with insomnia appears to be considerably less than that caused by someone with Obstructive Sleep Apnoea.[136]

While some qualitative work indicates that many couples attempt to resolve problems such as discordance in sleep,[137] the process of searching for a solution may lead to additional conflicts. Couples with discordant sleep schedules, therefore, may be exposed to high levels of stress which can impair sleep and lead to mental health problems.[138] Thus, couple-level sleep can affect individual sleep and mental health outcomes through a series of stress processes.[139] Couples, therefore, often modify their sleep/wake behaviours, for instance, women in co-sleeping couples may alter their bedtime or wake time to match their partners', contributing to longer total sleep time.[140] Additionally, they may fall asleep more easily due to the stress-relieving feelings of comfort and security gained by sleeping beside their partner.[141]

When couples are sleep concordant, they may perceive their sleep as subjectively better[142] due to feelings of security, despite increases in movements and disturbances.[143] Persons with a secure attachment style form and keep high-quality, close relationships.[144] They are able to use their partner as a secure base, from which they gain feelings of safety and protection, buffering against stress from the day, reducing psychological and physiological arousal, making sleep onset easier, and contributing to sounder sleep.[145] Thus, it is hypothesized that there will be a positive association between sleep concordance and sleep quality for people with greater attachment security.

However, not all couples experience such feelings of security from their partners. Individuals with insecure attachment are unable to use their partner as a secure base, and may not receive the stress-buffering, secure feelings normally associated with sleeping beside a partner.[146] For example, persons with avoidant attachment are uncomfortable with intimacy and prefer to be self-reliant rather than seek support from others,[147] suggesting that sleep concordance may have little benefit for them. Persons with anxious-ambivalent attachment experience chronic doubts about whether their partners reciprocate their romantic feelings and whether they are trustworthy. They can also view themselves as unworthy of love and are difficult to comfort and reassure.[148] The implication again is that sleep concordance may offer little benefit for sleep quality. Thus, it is expected that there will be little or no association between sleep concordance and sleep quality among individuals with greater attachment insecurity.

Attachment

Sleep is a vulnerable state that is antithetical to vigilance.[149] People need to feel safe and secure to be able to reduce vigilance, relax and fall asleep.[150] According to attachment theory, romantic partners serve as an important source for feelings of safety and security,[151] especially during times of vulnerability.

For example, in a study of 15 young heterosexual couples, Spiegelhalder et al.[152] investigated the importance of location and co-sleeping. They studied the participants under four separate conditions (a) both partners slept in the bed of the male; (b) both partners slept in the bed of the female; (c) each partner slept on his or her own in his or her own bed; (d) each partner slept on his or her own in the bed of the respective partner. Overall, their results suggest that sleep location does not appear to have a consistent and robust effect on sleep quantity or quality. However, the social setting did affect heterosexual young men, who were found to sleep longer and rise later when co-sleeping with their partner. In contrast, there was no significant effect of the social setting on sleep continuity parameters in women. In both sexes, sleep quality was perceived to be better when sleeping in pairs. However, there was a higher concordance of the partners' body movements on co-sleeping nights compared to the sleeping alone condition. This perhaps suggests that there is a perception of better sleep that is not necessarily borne out by the actuality.

Elsey[153] investigated the association between couple sleep concordance and subjective sleep quality across different levels of attachment, security, and insecurity. Women who scored higher on the secure attachment style reported higher sleep quality. Women who scored higher on the avoidant attachment style reported lower sleep quality. Sleeping beside a partner may be particularly beneficial for the sleep of women who report lower levels of attachment security or higher levels of attachment insecurity. This may be because women with greater attachment security can rely on themselves and utilize their own coping skills; essentially, they don't need their partner beside them to feel safe and relaxed at night.[154] Women with less attachment security may be unable to turn off attachment-related worries and self-soothe; thus, they experience trouble falling asleep, and so they actually benefit from having their partner beside them in bed for feelings of security and relief.[155]

However, the presence of a romantic partner in the bed is associated with a decrease of the deep, restorative slow-wave sleep[156] and an increased number of body movements during the night,[157] with the latter being most likely due to movement synchrony between partners,[158] i.e., if one partner moves in the night the other partner tends to also move, (Interesting, these effects are also observed in non-human primates).[159]

Kent de Grey et al.[160] investigated 92 married heterosexual couples found that individuals attachment anxiety significantly predicted poorer quality of their own sleep. In contrast, high attachment anxiety in both spouses predicted improved sleep quality. When both spouses are anxiously attached, it may be that each is eager to have positive interactions with the other, such that bedtime provides a setting in which concerns about attachment are allayed by the presence of one's partner, resulting in improved sleep quality.

Whereas high attachment avoidance in both spouses was associated with poorer sleep quality. For couples high in avoidance, bedtime may make attachment-related concerns more salient, leading to poorer sleep quality. It may also be that in such couples, coping strategies employed throughout the day can no longer be used at bedtime, contributing to sleep difficulties. For example, spouses who have been avoiding each other during the day to forestall discussion of an important, controversial topic may be forced to broach the subject at bedtime, precipitating an argument.

Feelings of safety and security (or their absence) are particularly important for optimizing sleep in couple relationships. Several studies have shown that insecurity in close relationships (i.e., 'attachment anxiety') is an independent correlate of poor subjective sleep quality and decreased sleep depth in both women and men.[161]

A study[162] conducted in 2010 in 29 couples, found that lower sleep efficiency on just one night was associated with more negative interactions with partners the following day. However, this finding held only for men.

Discordance

Sleep discordance can lead to problems as mentioned above, as it has been hypothesised that sleep discordance deviates from the cultural norm of the "ideological code of American family", Smith[163] argues that in the United States and most Western societies, practices within the family remain quite traditional.[164] The dominant cultural norm expects that not only do married couples sleep together, but husbands and wives synchronize their sleep schedules. Maintaining a concordant sleep schedule is an important social interaction process that sustains older adults' family identities.[165] When there is a deviation from this norm, it suggests an adult's inability to be a good husband or a good wife.[166] Therefore, it has been suggested that discordant sleep among couples can negatively impact adults' self-mastery and lead to disconfirmation, i.e., invalidation, of their family identities and roles. Anxiety, negative emotions, psychological distress, and/or depression are often observed among individuals who have lower levels of self-mastery and who experience identity disconfirmation.[167] Therefore, discordance in couples' sleep, being a behaviour that 'deviates' from a cultural norm, can affect mental health and affects individual-level sleep.[169]

Sex

Satisfaction with sexual life has been found to correlate negatively with sleep disturbance, suggesting that couples who were satisfied with their sex life suffered from fewer sleep disturbances. Furthermore, participants reported a better mood when they had sex at night. Intimacy is known to alleviate stress,[168] and stress has a negative impact on sleep and thus may mediate the influence of sexual encounters on sleep.

Sleep and marital discord

Kiecolt-Glaser et al.[170] provide an excellent overview of sleep and marital discord.

Although married people sleep better than single people on average,[171] marital discord negatively affects sleep quality and quantity.[172] Those in more strained marriages report higher insomnia than those who are happily married.[173] Yang et al.[174] found that discord-induced sleep problems exacerbated conflict that can lead to longer-term marital dysfunction, to the extent that more sleep problems at baseline were related to a lower degree of lower marital quality four years later. Another study showed that more destructive and less constructive conflict resulted in a decline in actigraphy-assessed sleep quality and duration over one year.[175] On days when couple interactions were more negative, women experienced worse actigraphy-assessed sleep that night.[176] Moreover, the sleep-disruptive effects of marital discord seem to be contagious; husbands' poorer sleep also followed wives' reports of greater marital tension.[177]

Several studies have shown that sleep and relationship quality are bidirectional. For instance, Gordon and Chen[178] found that people experienced more conflict in their relationships following nights when they slept worse relative to their own average across a 2-week period. Both partners experienced a lower ratio of positive to negative affect and reduced empathic accuracy when one partner slept poorly. Conflicts were found to most likely to be resolved when both partners were well-rested.

Kane et al.[179] found that greater self-disclosure predicted better sleep for wives, but not for husbands. On days when couples disclosed their feelings, they enjoyed better sleep and fewer negative-mood-related sleep disruptions at night. In a 2007 study of 69 couples,[180] those couples who were receiving treatment for sleep disorders reported fewer disagreements each week compared to couples who were not receiving treatment.

However, the direction of effects may be gender-dependent. Hasler and Troxel[181] found that higher levels of female relationship satisfaction during the day predicted better sleep for both her and her partner that night. However, for males, better sleep at night predicted higher male, but not female, relationship satisfaction the next day. In 2017 in the first study to demonstrate that improving marital quality can have a measurable impact on insomnia, Troxel et al.[182] found that improvements in marital satisfaction were associated with a lower risk of insomnia at the 3-month follow-up; although they found this was only statistically significant for husbands. To explain their findings, they hypothesised that "Perhaps wives in non-distressed marriages who experience more sleep loss at night (either at onset or after onset) are engaging in conversation or sexual activity with their husbands, thus increasing husband marital satisfaction."

The link between marital discord and sleep exhibits a dose-response relationship: more destructive conflict elevates the risk for sleep disturbance, to the extent that those who experience prolonged aggression sleep worse than those subjected to less frequent violence.[183] Beyond conflict and discord, exposure to one's partner's stressors impacts sleep; for instance, partners slept worse on days when osteoarthritis patients had more severe pain, particularly those who felt close in the relationship.[184] For patients, negative mood led to worse sleep when partners responded to pain in hostile or overzealous ways.[185]

Sleep loss and poor sleep can intensify conflict. In a diary study, when men slept more poorly, they reported more negative interactions with their partners the next day.[186] Likewise, couples who slept poorly over 14 nights reported more daily conflict with their partners than those who reported better sleep quality.[187] Worse sleep also translated into more negative affect and less positive affect during a discussion about marital problems; moreover, the partners were less able to assess their emotions or those of their partner accurately. These studies show that one partner's poor sleep affects not only their own mood and empathic accuracy but also the partner's.

Relationships are thought to be linked to sleep quality due to its evolutionarily adaptive function of providing a safe context in which sleeping individuals were protected from predators and enemies by close others.[188] There have been several studies examining whether social relationships characterized by high levels of support and satisfaction predict better sleep quality.[189] Several studies have found that perceived support is linked to better subjective and objective sleep quality.[190] Similarly, Troxel et al.[191] found that greater perceived social support predicted less actigraphy-assessed wakefulness after sleep onset, an important aspect of sleep. Moreover, interpersonal negativity or strain has also been linked to sleep quality. In one such study, Brummett and colleagues[192] found that negative affect associated with caregiving predicted poorer sleep quality (in this case, including sleep latency, duration, sleep disturbances, daytime dysfunction, etc.). Such an association may be due to the ability of interpersonal stressors to exacerbate social-affective processes.[193]

Yorgason[194] showed that when a wife reports of sleeping longer on a given night relative to their study average were linked to increases in both the number of positive marital events reported on the next day. Additionally, on days when wives said they had had better sleep quality than their study average, they endorsed less adverse matrimonial events on that day. Husband reports of higher sleep quality were related to higher daily marital satisfaction. Specifically, increases in wife hours slept on a given day significantly predicted an increase in the number of positive marital events and marital satisfaction reported by their husband on that same day. Similarly, husband hours slept and sleep quality were positively associated with wife reports of positive marital events. Higher wife daily feeling rested was linked to less negative marital events reported by husbands. These findings indicated that marital events do indeed predict sleep with poorer marital interactions and mood linked with poorer sleep. In common with other studies,[195] this study showed that increases in sleep quality and feeling rested were correlated with positive and negative marital events and daily marital satisfaction. Moreover, the number of hours slept was significantly and positively related to marital outcomes.

Troxel et al.[196] in their 2009 study, found that women in a satisfying marriage experienced significantly fewer sleep problems than women in non-satisfying marriages.

Kent et al.[197] examined the links between relationships and sleep quality in terms of positivity and negativity in social ties. They found that supportive ties were related to better sleep quality, whereas aversive ties were related to poorer sleep quality. They also found that these effects on sleep were mediated by depression. Supportive ties were found to be related to better sleep quality. Ailshire and Burgard[198] also reported that aversive ties are related to poorer sleep. Maranges and McNulty[199] examined of 68 newlywed couples to investigate the implications of sleep for daily marital evaluations. They found that spouses were more satisfied on days after which they had slept for a longer period of time. Furthermore, sleep also buffered husbands', but not wives', marital satisfaction against the implications of negative specific evaluations— husbands were better able to remain more globally satisfied despite negative evaluations of specific aspects of the relationship on days following more sleep. Remaining satisfied with a close intimate relationship often requires self-regulation,[200] and self-regulatory resources appear to be functionally limited when experiencing poor sleep.[201] Nevertheless, sleep is one way to replenish these resources,[202] which suggests sleep may offer self-regulatory benefits to relationships.

Interestingly, Hasler and Troxel[203] hypothesises that there may be a lagged effect of sleep (2 or 3 days following), i.e., the number of hours slept may be less important in marriage relationships on a given day than on coming days.

Sleep and aggression

Studies have shown that conflict and aggression are more likely when romantic partners have poor-quality sleep.[204] Poor-quality sleep is generally associated with both physical and psychological aggression in dating couples[205] and married couples.[206] Studies have shown that sleep problems are linked to aggression in romantic relationships.[207] Women report that their abusive partners were more abusive following a night of poor-quality sleep.[208] Relationship conflicts are more likely the day after a night of poor-quality sleep.[209] Female college students are more likely to be physically and psychologically abusive toward their boyfriends if they have poor-quality sleep.[210] Poor self-reported sleep quality is associated with increases in the perpetration of psychological, marital aggression for both men and women.[211]

Sleep deprivation is associated with increased activity in the amygdala, which is linked to the intensity of the emotional experience, and decreased connectivity between the amygdala and the medial prefrontal cortex, which is needed to regulate responses to emotion.[212] Emotion is a major component of marital interactions, and the ability to identify and regulate emotions is a critical skill for healthy marriages.[213] Everyday experiences of anger and frustration in marriages may be intensified and poorly controlled in the context of sleep problems.[214] There are bidirectional associations between sleep problems and aggression, i.e. just as sleep problems may undermine the neurological bases of self-control and lead to aggressive behaviour, the experience of marital aggression may prevent couples from obtaining healthy sleep. According to the model of sleep and wake being antithetical,[215] people need to feel safe, secure, and relaxed to achieve sleep. High levels of anger are, therefore, incompatible with sleep. Similarly, worry and stress about relationships or fear of victimization may prevent feelings of safety and security required for sleep. There are numerous studies supporting the idea that marital conflict is a risk factor for poor sleep.[216] Sleep may play an important role in aggression because it supports the neurological mechanisms of self-control.

Rauer et al.[217] found that for both men and women, higher initial levels of psychological abuse and increases in psychological abuse over time predicted more significant sleep problems three years later. These findings are explained by the fact that sleep loss leads to amplified responses to negative emotional stimuli[218] as well as greater negative affect, such as increased anger.[219] Thus, individuals who sleep poorly may be prone to more frequently and more severely negatively react to problems in their relationships than if they had slept better. Sleep loss is also associated with reduced empathy and recognition of emotions;[220] thus, poor sleep may impede understanding between relationship partners, creating more opportunity for conflict. Also, reduced empathy is associated with more mis-communication and an enhanced willingness to retaliate during conflict;[221] suggesting that poor sleep may lead to more damaging conflict. Moreover, just one night of sleep loss has been found to impair problem-solving,[222] something perhaps vital for achieving conflict resolution.

Keller et al.[223] in a study of 342 married couples, investigated the associations between sleep problems and marital aggression. They found that sleep problems (total PSQI score, daytime dysfunction, and sleep disturbances) rather than for sleep duration undermine self-control and that this lowered self-control leads to an increase in physical and psychological aggression. Schlarb et al.[224] found that destructive fighting behaviour was associated with poorer sleep quality and other studies[225] have shown that sarcastic criticism, accusing the partner of something and casting aspersions are associated with less sleep quality and more daytime sleepiness. Gordon and Chen[226] found that a poor night's sleep leads to more destructive fighting and less accurate empathetic reactions.

All this can have profound consequences as shown by Birditt et al.[227] who reported that destructive fighting behaviour is related to a higher divorce rate.

Mental health and couple's sleep

In a study by Walters et al.[228] examined whether anxiety or depression symptoms predicted an individual's sleep or their bedpartner's sleep, in fifty-two bed-sharing couples where one partner experienced insomnia and in couples without sleep disorders. They found that higher anxiety symptoms predicted increased vulnerability to being woken by their bedpartner, as well as increased frequency of waking their bedpartner up during the night in patients with insomnia, but not in non-sleep-disordered couples.

Revenson et al.[229] showed that husbands' anxiety and depressive symptoms had a stronger effect on their wives' anxiety and depression than the other way around, but this was not moderated by one's own sleep duration. For both wives and husbands, higher levels of depressive symptoms and anxiety predicted shorter sleep duration for their partner one year later. However, the effect of husbands' mental health on their wives was again more substantial.

Physical effects of couple's sleep

Not only can emotional health be affected by sleeping as a couple can also compromise physical health, Uchino et al.[230] found significant evidence for partner's poor sleep (i.e., sleep disturbances, sleep latency) having an effect on one's own inflammatory outcomes. Wilson et al.[231] found that people who slept fewer hours in the past two nights had higher inflammatory responses following marital conflict than those who slept more. They also found that when both partners had slept less, they behaved more negatively and less positively during conflict. However, they were protected from short sleep's behavioural effects if one of the partners had sufficient sleep in the two previous nights. Furthermore, despite shorter sleep, couples who made greater use of emotion expression and cognitive reappraisal did not show increased stimulated cytokine production. These findings suggest that the risks of short sleep in daily life lie in heightened inflammatory sensitivity to stressors and that these risks depend on both partners' sleep and emotion regulation strategies. Those who slept fewer hours had higher levels of markers of inflammation, (for the scientifically minded among you, tumour necrosis factor alpha, (TNF-α) and interleukin-6 (IL-6)), after a marital problem discussion compared to their more rested counterparts. These results suggest that recent nights without sufficient sleep may promote a person's inflammatory responses to interpersonal conflict and perhaps other stressors.

Subjective insomnia symptoms among middle-aged and older adults in intimate partnerships are related to their heart disease risk. For example, Shih[232] examined data from 2010, 2012, and 2014 Health and Retirement Studies and found that insomnia symptoms measured at baseline were related to an increased risk for heart disease for husbands. Wives' insomnia was related to an increased risk of incident heart disease for husbands, but husbands' insomnia was not associated with wives' risk of heart disease.

Walters et al.[233] recent research has begun to consider the role of the bed partner, documenting how romantic bedsharing can be important for both sleep quality[234] and health.[235] Romantic couples have previously been shown to co-regulate levels of cortisol, blood pressure, and mood.[236] Relatively recent work shows co-regulation extends to sleep/wake states. Sleep/wake concordance has been used to describe covariation of sleep and wake states within bedsharing couples (i.e., whether individuals are both awake or asleep at the same time).[237] For example, in healthy controls, couples are in the same sleep/ wake state for 75% of the night[238], and one-third of couples' night-time wrist movements occur in synchrony, suggesting a third of all wake after sleep onset is common between partners.[239] Levels of sleep/wake concordance decreased with increasing age and relationship length.[240] Effects of bedsharing may also depend on sex,[241] with females demonstrating compromised objective sleep efficiency (SE) when co-sleeping compared with sleeping alone,[242] and males exhibiting longer total sleep time (TST) when co-sleeping.[243]

The association between sleep-wake concordance and health outcomes are more robust for women.[244] This sex differences may be explained by the evolutionary reliance of women on men due to their size and dominance for protection from potential predators.[245] Perhaps the beneficial feelings of security women gain by sleeping beside their partner are not shared by men. Additionally, men may not be as impacted by environmental and relational influences as women when trying to fall asleep.[246]

APPENDIX 2

Tips and techniques that may help you get better sleep

You may have negotiated the minefield of your sleeping arrangements and have your own luxurious sleep sanctuary, but neither Jennifer nor I would claim that these automatically guarantee a good sleep. There can be many causes of poor sleep and while some people have serious problems with their sleep that necessitates the intervention of their GP, for most people suffering from poor sleep there are many things they can do for themselves to improve their sleep.

Pretty much every piece of modern sleep self-help literature, however 'new and revolutionary' they claim to be, has at its core called the concept of 'sleep hygiene'; (based on Hauri's "Rules of Sleep Hygiene" which were published in the early 1977[247]). Over the years these so-called 'rules' have been endlessly repeated, expanded and modified by various authors. However, we are all individual so a 'one size fits all' set of rules cannot be expected to work for everyone. Everyone wants the 'Top 10 Tips' for a good night's sleep as though there really were 10 magic rules that will help everyone sleep, unfortunately this is not the case.

To get better sleep it is important for you to find your own individual way to sleep. There are not '10 top tips' but 3 general principles: –

The most important things to have in order to get better sleep:

- A quiet mind. "All worry and vexatious circumstances should as far as possible be habitually excluded from the mind for a considerable time before the regular hour of retiring." J. Leonard Corning, Brain Rest 1885[248]
- A relaxed body. "Before going to bed, the body ought to be brought into that state which gives us the surest chance of relapsing speedily into sleep." Robert Macnish, The Anatomy of Sleep 1830[249]
- A bedroom conducive to sleep.

Anything that helps you achieve a quiet mind and relaxed body will help you sleep. Thus, as an individual you need to find your own way to sleep whatever that may be. Remember the adage – one man's relaxation is another man's stress. However, people always want affirmation as to whether what they do works and so I often get asked questions like;

Q   Does camomile tea help you sleep?

A   If you like the taste and feel more relaxed for having drunk it, YES

Q   Does yoga help you sleep?

A   If it is relaxing for you, YES

Q   Does thinking of different animals starting with each letter of the alphabet help you sleep?

A   If you find this relaxing, YES

You should by now see a pattern,

Q   Does XXXX help you sleep?

A   If YOU find it relaxing, YES

But as you are no doubt aware you can be physically exhausted but still not sleep because your mind is racing and so while a relaxed body is important a quiet mind is a prerequisite for sleep.

There is some very general guidance that may point you towards what may best work for you. The first step is to look at your life and lifestyle to see if there are things that may be causing your poor sleep, e.g., diet, exercise patterns, sleeping environment, personal habits, lifestyle, stress and worries of daily living. Keep in mind that good sleep doesn't just happen; to go to sleep, you need to quieten your mind and relax your body.

During the day

The best way to get a good night sleep is to be awake

during the day. Daytime exercise, both physical and mental, can promote good sleep. It is also important to get adequate exposure to natural light during the day, as this is the major signal to the brain that it is time to be awake.

Going to bed

Go to bed when you are sleepy, not when the TV programme you are watching finishes. Most people's preparation for sleep seems to involve nothing more than turning the TV off, having a pee, brushing their teeth and then getting into bed and expecting to fall asleep, then being surprised that it does not happen. Thus, one of the most important things you can do is to establish a regular relaxing bedtime routine. This will signal to the body that it is time for sleep and will allow you to put the stresses and worries of the day behind you. You should spend at least 30 minutes winding down before bed this means turning the TV/computer off and doing those things that help you quieten the mind and relax your body; so, don't work, don't argue with your partner, don't open the gas bill etc. Once you are in bed because you are relaxed, you should gently drift off to sleep. It is important that you don't try to fall asleep, the harder you try, the more worked up you will get because you aren't falling asleep, so the less likely you are to actually fall asleep.

The bedroom

The bedroom should be a sanctuary reserved for sleep and thus, the sleep environment needs to be pleasant and relaxing (get rid of the TV and computers, etc.). It should also be dark, (either use heavy curtains or eyeshades) and it should be as quiet as possible, (if this is difficult then consider using the earplugs now available which are comfortable to sleep in). The bedroom should not be stuffy, fresh air is good for sleep and it should be neither too hot nor cold. Finally, the bed should be very comfortable and as big as you can fit into your bedroom.

During the night

If you are tossing and turning for more than 30 minutes at the start of the night or 20 minutes during the night, it may be helpful to get out of bed, or switch the light on, and do something else, only going back to bed when you feel sleepy again. If you still don't fall asleep again, get up, do something else and go back to bed when you are sleepy—lying in bed trying to fall asleep and getting ever more frustrated that you don't is not conducive to falling back to sleep.

In the morning

The body craves regularity and so having a regular wake up time can be a very positive change. This is because the body starts preparing to wake up about one and a half hours before you actually awake. Therefore, if your body knows when it is going to wake, then it can maximise the sleep opportunity as well as prepare itself to wake up, however, if it does not know when you are going to wake it cannot prepare and thus you are liable to feel groggy when you wake.

Think guidance, not law

Sleep is a very individual thing and so the sleep hygiene 'rules' should be seen merely as guidance that needs personal adaptation – listen to your body. So, whilst the 'rules' says one thing, think about the way YOUR life really is. Some examples

Avoid stimulants such as caffeine, nicotine, and alcohol too close to bedtime.
- But remember that although alcohol in itself can disturb sleep, sometimes perhaps the relaxation gained from sipping a fine single malt in front of a roaring fire outweigh the possible effects of the alcohol for some individuals?
- But if you have had a lovely three-course meal with friends and a few glasses of wine, then why not round off the evening with a nice cup of coffee, the food and drink are probably going to disturb your sleep, so one coffee is not really going to make much difference.
- If you have been regularly drinking 2 cups of black coffee just before bed for many years and you have only now developed a sleep problem it is almost certain the coffee is not the cause of the problem.

Associate your bed with sleep. It's not a good idea to use

your bed to watch TV, listen to the radio, or read.

- But if reading or listening to the radio/TV is part of your wind-down then use it as just that, for many reading in bed is an essential sleep inducer.

Don't smoke before going to bed – nicotine is a stimulant and will keep you awake.

- However, remember that for some people, nicotine withdrawal overnight could also disturb sleep.

Basically, look at your life and find those things that will help you to quieten your mind and relax your body.

Remember you cannot find sleep – you have to let sleep find you.

References

1. https://www.female.com.au/sleeping-apart-not-falling-apart.htm
2. https://www.huffpost.com/entry/jennifer-adams-sleeping-apart_n_3751489?
   https://www.youtube.com/watch?v=gVE5TEmhz2A
   https://www.chicagotribune.com/lifestyles/sc-couples-sleeping-apart-family-1027-20151020-story.html
   https://www.couriermail.com.au/questnews/logan/dedicated-separate-sleeper-and-author-jennifer-adams-says-couples-can-sleep-apart-and-be-happy/news-story/8d5b9d9ffb653dd023eff0daef6db68c
   https://www.youtube.com/watch?v=5zFNNqqArY0
   https://www.dailymail.co.uk/femail/article-5663175/Happily-married-couple-Jennifer-Adams-Fraser-Mackay-not-shared-bed-nearly-14-YEARS.html
3. http://news.bbc.co.uk/1/hi/health/5197440.stm
4. https://www.dailymail.co.uk/femail/article-1173803/Separate-beds-28-Why-loving-couple-want-sleep-apart.html
   http://news.bbc.co.uk/1/hi/health/8245578.stm
   https://www.dailymail.co.uk/sciencetech/article-1212127/Sharing-bed-bad-health-Want-dream-marriage-Then-sleep-separate-beds.html

https://www.dailymail.co.uk/femail/article-1222936/How--Get-good-nights-sleep.html

https://www.psychologytoday.com/us/blog/sleep-newzzz/200912/the-secret-happy-marriage-and-healthy-self-separate-beds-i-doubt-it

https://www.dailymail.co.uk/femail/article-1303935/More-couples-opting-separate-bedrooms--surprising-results.html

https://www.telegraph.co.uk/news/science/6157455/Sleeping-with-your-partner-could-be-bad-for-your-health.html

https://www.abc.net.au/news/2009-09-10/sleeping-alone-the-answer-to-a-good-night/1424894

https://www.express.co.uk/expressyourself/109752/Why-I-d-rather-sleep-well-than-sleep-together

5. Evalyn Waugh. Vile Bodies, Chapman & Hall 1930

6. Dittami, J., Keckeis, M., Machatschke, I., Katina, S., Zeitlhofer, J., & Kloesch, G. (2007). Sex differences in the reactions to sleeping in pairs versus sleeping alone in humans. Sleep and Biological Rhythms, 5(4), 271-276.

7. Klösch, G., with Dittami, J., and Zeitlhofer, J. Sleeping better together, Hunter House Inc., Canada, 2011, p2

8. Rosenblatt, P. C., Two in a Bed: The Social System of Couple Bed Sharing, State University of New York Press, NY, 2006, p13

9. http://today.ninemsn.com.au/article.aspx?id=7947365

10. http://www.washingtonpost.com/wp-dyn/content/article/2006/01/09/AR2006010901549.html

11. https://qz.com/quartzy/1553076/choosing-to-sleep-in-separate-beds-is-the-last-relationship-taboo/

12. Esther Perel Mating in Captivity: Reconciling the Erotic and the Domestic by HarperCollins Publishers Sept. 2006

13. http://www.funfactz.com/tv-facts/the-first-couple-to-be-shown-in-bed-1734.html

14. http://www.snopes.com/radiotv/tv/marykay.asp

15. http://www.imdb.com/title/tt0043208/trivia

16. http://www.spaceandculture.org/2007/03/15/rewriting-marriage-two-beds-bedrooms-at-a-time/

17. http://www.huffingtonpost.com/josey-vogels/couples-sleep-separately_b_1212775.html

18. http://www.dailymail.co.uk/home/you/article-475998/Why-bed-

hopping-save-marriage.html

19. http://medcitynews.com/2013/09/sleep-apart-stay-together-separate-bedrooms-better-couples/

20. http://www.guardian.co.uk/world/2007/mar/12/usa.richardluscombe

21. https://sleepstandards.com/

22. Klösch, G., with Dittami, J., and Zeitlhofer, J. Sleeping better together, Hunter House Inc., Canada, 2011, p5 & p 27

23. Klösch, G., with Dittami, J., and Zeitlhofer, J. Sleeping better together, Hunter House Inc., Canada, 2011, p35

24. http://women.timesonline.co.uk/tol/life_and_style/women/relationships/article6008921.ece

25. For more see this book - Bundling: its origin, progress, and decline in America by Henry Reed Stiles 1871 https://ia801409.us.archive.org/6/items/bundlingitsorigi00stil/bundlingitsorigi00stil.pdf

26. http://www.mynippon.com/romance/married.htm

27. http://en.rocketnews24.com/2013/12/05/two-people-two-beds-why-do-so-many-japanese-spouses-sleep-separately/

28. http://en.wikipedia.org/wiki/Marriage

29. Klösch, G., with Dittami, J., and Zeitlhofer, J. Sleeping better together, Hunter House Inc., Canada, 2011, p74

30. http://www.jewfaq.org/sex.htm

31. http://www.islamswomen.com/marriage/fiqh_of_marriage_9.php; http://quod.lib.umich.edu/k/koran/ (4:34)

32. Hilary Hinds, A Cultural History of Twin Beds, Routledge; 2019

33. http://www.vanityfair.com/society/2012/01/queen-elizabeth-201201

34. http://www.dailymail.co.uk/news/article-1315348/Prince-Michael-Kent-admits-wife-spend-lot-time-apart-dismisses-marriage-rumours.html; http://www.dailymail.co.uk/news/article-2458334/Princess-Michael-Kent-horror-having-downsize.html

35. http://ohnotheydidnt.livejournal.com/70070135.html

36. http://www.huffingtonpost.com/2012/06/27/celebrity-sleep-separate-beds_n_1632239.html

37. https://www.celebitchy.com/382364/baz_luhrmann_says_separate_bedrooms_saved_his_marriage_makes_sense/

38. https://www.independent.co.uk/news/people/news/couples-

together-apart-were-closejust-not-that-close-2110286.html

39. https://inews.co.uk/opinion/gwyneth-paltrow-brad-falchuk-marriage-living-separately-unconventional-193113

40. https://meaww.com/sandra-bullock-boyfriend-bryan-randall-sleep-separate-beds-relationship-different-lifestyles
For other perhaps less famous people who sleep separately see for instance https://www.dailymail.co.uk/tvshowbiz/article-8238821/Suranne-Jones-husband-make-sure-good-nights-slumber-sleeping-separate-beds.html;
https://people.com/tv/carson-daly-jokes-wife-siri-may-never-sleep-together-again-after-sleep-divorcing-last-year/
https://www.thethings.com/20-little-known-facts-about-tom-brady-and-gisele-bundchens-relationship/
https://www.heart.co.uk/lifestyle/parenting/sam-faiers-boyfriend-paul-sleep-separate-rooms/
https://www.express.co.uk/celebrity-news/1231604/chris-evans-virgin-radio-wife-natasha-shishmanian-family-children-latest
https://www.mirror.co.uk/3am/celebrity-news/scarlett-moffatt-admits-new-boyfriend-20668246
https://uk.news.yahoo.com/billy-connolly-and-wife-pamela-stephenson-now-need-separate-beds-because-of-parkinsons-disease-effects-092511782.html
https://www.dailymail.co.uk/femail/article-4287692/Edwina-Bartholomew-says-sleeps-separately-partner.html
https://metro.co.uk/2019/09/15/fearne-cotton-wont-share-bed-husband-jesse-wood-case-wakes-10746430/

41. Taylor, B., 'Unconsciousness and Society: The Sociology of Sleep', International Journal of Politics, Culture and Society, 1993; vol. 6, no. 3, pp 463–471

42. https://metro.co.uk/2018/04/05/try-sleep-divorce-7442927/
https://globalnews.ca/news/4039314/sleeping-apart-good-for-marriage/
https://www.independent.co.uk/life-style/sleep-divorce-americans-partner-separate-beds-mattress-clarity-study-us-a8275631.html
https://www.insider.com/what-is-sleep-divorce-relationship-trick-2018-4
https://www.psychologytoday.com/gb/blog/between-you-and-

me/201912/should-you-be-considering-sleep-divorce
https://www.nytimes.com/2019/07/31/fashion/weddings/is-it-time-for-a-sleep-divorce.html
https://www.theatlantic.com/entertainment/archive/2019/11/sleep-divorce-bedroom-splitting-night/602122/

43. 3 x Carlin: An Orgy of George including Brain Droppings, Napalm and Silly Putty, and When Will Jesus Bring the Pork Chops? Hachette UK 2015

44. http://plato.stanford.edu/entries/alcmaeon/>

45. http://www.better-sleep-better-life.com/benefits-of-sleep.html; http://longevity.about.com/od/lifelongenergy/tp/healthy_sleep.htm

46. http://www.uptodate.com/contents/classification-of-sleep-disorders

47. Klösch, G., with Dittami, J., and Zeitlhofer, J. sleeping better together, Hunter House Inc., Canada, 2011, p35

48. Dittami, J., Keckeis, M., Machatschke, I., Katina, S., Zeitlhofer, J., & Kloesch, G. (2007). Sex differences in the reactions to sleeping in pairs versus sleeping alone in humans. Sleep and Biological Rhythms, 5(4), 271-276.

49. Klösch, G., with Dittami, J., and Zeitlhofer, J. sleeping better together, Hunter House Inc., Canada, 2011, p75

50. http://www.sealysleepcensus.com.au/docs/SleepCensus FinalReportApril2012.pdf

51. http://www.sleepfoundation.org/article/press-release/annual-sleep-america-poll-exploring-connections-communications-technology-use-

52. http://www.anzca.edu.au/resources/professional-documents/documents/professional-standards/professional-standards-43.html

53. https://www.optalert.com/how-fatigue-played-a-role-in-some-of-the-worlds-biggest-disasters/

54. http://www.abc.net.au/unleashed/167376.html

55. http://www.apa.org/topics/sleep/why.aspx?item=1

56. http://health.howstuffworks.com/mental-health/sleep/basics/sleep-obesity.htm

57. http://www.abc.net.au/catalyst/stories/2987827.htm

58. Klösch, G., with Dittami, J., and Zeitlhofer, J. Sleeping better

together, Hunter House Inc., Canada, 2011, p39

59. http://www.ucsf.edu/news/2009/08/4281/first-human-gene-implicated-regulating-length-human-sleep

60. Consensus Conference Panel, Watson, N. F., Badr, M. S., Belenky, G., Bliwise, D. L., Buxton, O. M., ... & Tasali, E. (2015). Recommended amount of sleep for a healthy adult: a joint consensus statement of the American Academy of Sleep Medicine and Sleep Research Society. Journal of Clinical Sleep Medicine, 11(6), 591-592.

61. Benjamin Franklin. Poor Richard's Almanack 1735 edition.

62. American Academy of Sleep Medicine. "Wives' sleep problems have negative impact on marital interactions, study finds." ScienceDaily. ScienceDaily, 14 June 2011.

63. American Academy of Sleep Medicine. "Poor Sleep Is Associated With Lower Relationship Satisfaction In Both Women And Men." ScienceDaily. ScienceDaily, 15 June 2009.

64. Larson, J.H., Crane, D.R. and Smith, C.W., 1991. Morning and night couples: the effect of wake and sleep patterns on marital adjustment. Journal of Marital and Family Therapy, 17(1), pp.53-65.

65. Inside Mr Ender, William Heinemann 1963

66. Rosenblatt, P. C., Two in a Bed: The Social System of Couple Bed Sharing, State University of New York Press, NY, 2006,

67. Beninati, W., Harris, C. D., Herold, D. L., & Shepard Jr, J. W. (1999, October). The effect of snoring and obstructive sleep apnea on the sleep quality of bed partners. In Mayo Clinic Proceedings (Vol. 74, No. 10, pp. 955-958). Elsevier.

68. Rosenblatt, P. C., Two in a Bed: The Social System of Couple Bed Sharing, State University of New York Press, NY, 2006, p13

69. http://www.industrialnoisecontrol.com/comparative-noise-examples.htm

70. http://www.powells.com/biblio?show=0553587129&page=excerpt

71. http://www.dailymail.co.uk/news/article-1220595/Meet-grandmother-snores-111-decibels--louder-JET-plane.html

72. http://hearing-protection.4ursafety.com/articles.html

73. http://www.industrialnoisecontrol.com/comparative-noise-examples.htm

74. http://en.wikipedia.org/wiki/John_Wesley_Hardin

75. http://www.dailymail.co.uk/health/article-2110674/How-stop-husband-wife-wrecking-nights-sleep-snoring.html

76. http://www.thetimes.co.uk/tto/health/article1963959.ece

77. Baker, F. C., & Driver, H. S. (2007). Circadian rhythms, sleep, and the menstrual cycle. Sleep medicine, 8(6), 613-622.

78. Groeger, J.A., Zijlstra, F.R.H. and Dijk, D.J., 2004. Sleep quantity, sleep difficulties and their perceived consequences in a representative sample of some 2000 British adults. Journal of sleep research, 13(4), pp.359-371.

79. Shepard, J.W., 2002. Pets and sleep Sleep Vol. 25, pp. A520

80. http://www.sleepsurvey.net.au/the-sleep-survey/results/

81. http://www.sealysleepcensus.com.au/docs/SleepCensusFinal ReportApril2012.pdf

82. http://uninews.cqu.edu.au/UniNews/currentEdition.do

83. http://archive.supermarketguru.com/page.cfm/30169

84. http://www.sleepsurvey.net.au/the-sleep-survey/results/

85. http://www.apa.org/topics/sleep/why.aspx?item=1

86. http://www.sealysleepcensus.com.au/docs/SleepCensusFinal ReportApril2012.pdf

87. Salmela, T., Colley, A., & Häkkilä, J. (2019, May). Together in Bed? Couples' Mobile Technology Use in Bed. In Proceedings of the 2019 CHI Conference on Human Factors in Computing Systems (pp. 1-12).

88. http://www.sleepfoundation.org/sites/default/files/ sleepinamericapoll/ SIAP_2011_Summary_of_Findings.pdf

89. Tazawa, Y., & Okada, K. (2001). Physical signs associated with excessive television-game playing and sleep deprivation. Pediatrics International, 43(6), 647-650.

    Van den Bulck, J. (2003). Text messaging as a cause of sleep interruption in adolescents, evidence from a cross-sectional study. Journal of Sleep Research, 12(3), pp.263-263.

    Van den Bulck, J. (2004). Television viewing, computer game playing, and Internet use and self-reported time to bed and time out of bed in secondary-school children. Sleep, 27(1), 101-104.

90. http://www.dailymail.co.uk/sciencetech/article-2178090/Too-light-night-causes-depression.html

91. Meadows R, Venn S, Hislop J, Stanley N, Arber S. (2005) Investigating couples' sleep: an evaluation of actigraphic analysis

techniques. Journal of Sleep Research 14 377-386

92. http://www.sleepfoundation.org/article/sleep-america-polls/2005-adult-sleep-habits-and-styles

93. Phineas Finn St Paul's Magazine October 1867 to May 1868

94. Hislop, J. and Arber, S. (2003c). Sleep as a social act: A window on gender roles and relationships. S. Arber, K. Davidson and J. Ginn. (eds) Gender & Ageing: Changing Roles and Relationships, Maidenhead: McGraw Hill/Open University Press, 186-205.

95. Hislop, J. (2007). A bed of roses or a bed of thorns? Negotiating the couple relationship through sleep. Sociological Research Online, 12(5), 146-158.

96. Stone, D., Patton, B., & Heen, S., Difficult Conversations: How to Discuss What Matters Most, Penguin Books, New York, NY, 2010

97. Bradbury, T., Karney, B. Intimate Relationships, Norton W. W. & Company Inc, New York, NY 2010

98. http://www.ehow.com/feature_12158549_two-beds-better-one.html

99. Klösch, G., with Dittami, J., and Zeitlhofer, J. Sleeping better together, Hunter House Inc., Canada, 2011, p52

100. http://www.independent.ie/lifestyle/independent-woman/health-fitness/is-sleeping-the-new-sex-1766358.html

101. http://www.harpyness.com/2011/01/31/on-living-together-but-sleeping-separately/

102. Coontz, S., A Strange Stirring: The Feminine Mystique and American Women at the Dawn of the 1960s, Basic Books, New York, NY, 2011

103. Gordon, A. M., & Chen, S. (2014). The role of sleep in interpersonal conflict: do sleepless nights mean worse fights? Social Psychological and Personality Science, 5(2), 168-175.

104. Hasler, B. P., & Troxel, W. M. (2010). Couples' nighttime sleep efficiency and concordance: Evidence for bidirectional associations with daytime relationship functioning. Psychosomatic medicine, 72(8), 794.

105. Larson, J. H., Crane, D. R., & Smith, C. W. (1991). Morning and night couples: the effect of wake and sleep patterns on marital adjustment. Journal of Marital and Family Therapy, 17(1), 53-65.

106. https://www.esquire.com/entertainment/interviews/a2053/esq0102-jan-fisher/

107. Impett, E. A., Gable, S. L., & Peplau, L. A. (2005). Giving up and giving in: The costs and benefits of daily sacrifice in intimate relationships. Journal of personality and social psychology, 89(3), 327.

108. Gable, S. L. (2006). Approach and avoidance social motives and goals. Journal of personality, 74(1), 175-222.

109. Dressler, L., Consensus Through Conversation: How to Achieve High-Commitment Decisions, Berrett-Koehler Publishers, San Fransisco, 2006

110. Hislop, J. (2007). A bed of roses or a bed of thorns? Negotiating the couple relationship through sleep. Sociological Research Online, 12(5), 146-158.

111. Hislop, J., & Arber, S. (2003). Sleepers wake! The gendered nature of sleep disruption among mid-life women. Sociology, 37(4), 695-711.

112. http://www.gottman.com/49847/The-Love-Lab.html

113. To a Mouse, on Turning Her Up in Her Nest With the Plough, November, 1785"

114. Dennis Gabor "Inventing the Future" 1963

115. Klösch, G., with Dittami, J., and Zeitlhofer, J. Sleeping better together, Hunter House Inc., Canada, 2011, p122

116. http://healthysleep.med.harvard.edu/healthy/science/how/external-factors

117. http://online.wsj.com/article/SB2000142405274870384660457544 7380187007528.html

118. http://www.thehappinessinstitute.com/

119. http://bottomlinepublications.com/content/drafts/sleep-apart-grow-closer/print?tmpl=component

120. http://www.quotationspage.com/quote/1990.html

121. J. L. Elkhorne. Edison — The Fabulous Drone, in 73 Vol. XLVI, No. 3 (March 1967), p. 52

122. The Soul of Man 1891

123. http://en.wikipedia.org/wiki/Maslow's_hierarchy_of_needs

124. http://www.nytimes.com/2007/03/11/us/11separate.html?_r=2&oref=slogin&

125. Klösch, G., with Dittami, J., and Zeitlhofer, J. Sleeping better together, Hunter House Inc., Canada, 2011, p144

126. Lauderdale D. S., Philip Schumm L., Kurina L. M., McClintock M.,

Thisted R. A., Chen J. H., & Waite L. (2014). Assessment of sleep in the National Social Life, Health, and Aging Project. The Journals of Gerontology, Series B: Psychological Sciences and Social Sciences, 69(Suppl. 2), S125–S133.

127. Pankhurst, F. P., & Home, J. A. (1994). The influence of bed partners on movement during sleep. Sleep, 17(4), 308-315.

128. Meadows, R., Venn, S., Hislop, J., Stanley, N., & Arber, S. (2005). Investigating couples' sleep: an evaluation of actigraphic analysis techniques. Journal of Sleep Research, 14(4), 377-386.

129. Gunn, H. E., Buysse, D. J., Hasler, B. P., Begley, A., & Troxel, W. M. (2015). Sleep concordance in couples is associated with relationship characteristics. Sleep, 38(6), 933-939.

130. Chen, J. H. (2018). Couples' sleep and psychological distress: A dyadic perspective. The Journals of Gerontology: Series B, 73(1), 30-39.

131. Pearlin, L. I. (1989). The sociological study of stress. Journal of Health and Social Behavior, 30, 241–256.
Pearlin, L. I. (2010). The life course and the stress process: Some conceptual comparisons. The Journals of Gerontology, Series B: Psychological Sciences and Social Sciences, 65, 207–215

132. Pearlin, L. I., Schieman, S., Fazio, E. M., & Meersman, S. C. (2005). Stress, health, and the life course: Some conceptual perspectives. Journal of Health and Social Behavior, 46, 205–219.

133. Rosenblatt, P. C. (2006). Two in a bed: The social system of couple bed sharing. Albany, NY: SUNY Press.

134. Lee, S., Martire, L. M., Damaske, S. A., Mogle, J. A., Zhaoyang, R., Almeida, D. M., & Buxton, O. M. (2018). Covariation in couples' nightly sleep and gender differences. Sleep health, 4(2), 201-208.

135. Walters, E. M., Phillips, A. J., Mellor, A., Hamill, K., Jenkins, M. M., Norton, P. J., & Drummond, S. P. (2020). Sleep and wake are shared and transmitted between individuals with insomnia and their bed-sharing partners. Sleep, 43(1), zsz206.

136. Henry, D., & Rosenthal, L. (2013). "Listening for his breath:" The significance of gender and partner reporting on the diagnosis, management, and treatment of obstructive sleep apnea. Social science & medicine, 79, 48-56.
Monroe, L. J. (1967). Psychological and physiological differences between good and poor sleepers. Journal of abnormal psychology,

72(3), 255.

137. Hislop, J., & Arber, S. (2003). Sleepers wake! The gendered nature of sleep disruption among mid-life women. Sociology, 37, 695–711.
Meadows, R., Arber, S., Venn, S., & Hislop, J. (2008). Engaging with sleep: Male definitions, understandings and attitudes. Sociology of Health & Illness, 30, 696–710.

138. Akerstedt, T. (2006). Psychosocial stress and impaired sleep. Scandinavian Journal of Work, Environment & Health, 32, 493–501.
Lorant, V., Deliège, D., Eaton, W., Robert, A., Philippot, P., & Ansseau, M. (2003). Socioeconomic inequalities in depression: A meta-analysis. American Journal of Epidemiology, 157, 98– 112.

139. Pearlin, L. I. (1989). The sociological study of stress. Journal of Health and Social Behavior, 30, 241–256.
Pearlin, L. I., Schieman, S., Fazio, E. M., & Meersman, S. C. (2005). Stress, health, and the life course: Some conceptual perspectives. Journal of Health and Social Behavior, 46, 205–219.

140. Meadows, R., Venn, S., Hislop, J., Stanley, N., & Arber, S. (2005). Investigating couples' sleep: an evaluation of actigraphic analysis techniques. Journal of Sleep Research, 14(4), 377-386.

141. Troxel, W. M., Buysse, D. J., Hall, M., & Matthews, K. A. (2009). Marital happiness and sleep disturbances in a multi-ethnic sample of middle- aged women. Behavioral Sleep Medicine, 7, 2–19.
Troxel, W. M. (2010). It's more than sex: Exploring the dyadic nature of sleep and implications for health. Psychosomatic medicine, 72(6), 578.

142. Richter, K., Adam, S., Geiss, L., Peter, L., & Niklewski, G. (2016). Two in a bed: The influence of couple sleeping and chronotypes on relationship and sleep. An overview. Chronobiology International, 33, 1464– 1472.

143. Pankhurst, F. P., & Home, J. A. (1994). The influence of bed partners on movement during sleep. Sleep, 17(4), 308-315.

144. Bartholomew, K. (1990). Avoidance of intimacy: An attachment perspective. Journal of Social and Personal relationships, 7(2), 147-178.

145. Sbarra, D. A., & Hazan, C. (2008). Coregulation, dysregulation, self-regulation: An integrative analysis and empirical agenda for understanding adult attachment, separation, loss, and recovery.

Personality and Social Psychology Review, 12(2), 141-167.

Troxel, W. M., Buysse, D. J., Hall, M., & Matthews, K. A. (2009). Marital happiness and sleep disturbances in a multi-ethnic sample of middle- aged women. Behavioral Sleep Medicine, 7, 2–19.

Troxel, W. M. (2010). It's more than sex: Exploring the dyadic nature of sleep and implications for health. Psychosomatic medicine, 72(6), 578.

146. Troxel, W. M., Buysse, D. J., Hall, M., & Matthews, K. A. (2009). Marital happiness and sleep disturbances in a multi-ethnic sample of middle- aged women. Behavioral Sleep Medicine, 7, 2–19.

147. Sbarra, D. A., & Hazan, C. (2008). Coregulation, dysregulation, self-regulation: An integrative analysis and empirical agenda for understanding adult attachment, separation, loss, and recovery. Personality and Social Psychology Review, 12(2), 141-167.

148. Sbarra, D. A., & Hazan, C. (2008). Coregulation, dysregulation, self-regulation: An integrative analysis and empirical agenda for understanding adult attachment, separation, loss, and recovery. Personality and Social Psychology Review, 12, 141–167

149. Dahl, R. E. (1996). The regulation of sleep and arousal: Development and psychopathology. Development and Psychopathology, 8, 3–27

150. Troxel, W. M. (2010). It's more than sex: Exploring the dyadic nature of sleep and implications for health. Psychosomatic medicine, 72(6), 578.

151. Hazan, C., & Shaver, P. R. (1987). Romantic love conceptualized as an attachment process. Journal of Personality and Social Psychology, 52, 511–524.

152. Spiegelhalder, K., Regen, W., Siemon, F., Kyle, S. D., Baglioni, C., Feige, B., Riemann, D. (2016). Your place or mine? Does the sleep location matter in young couples? Behavioral Sleep Medicine, 15, 1–9.

153. Elsey, T., Keller, P. S., & El-Sheikh, M. (2019). The role of couple sleep concordance in sleep quality: Attachment as a moderator of associations. Journal of sleep research, 28(5), e12825.

154. Carmichael, C. L., & Reis, H. T. (2005). Attachment, sleep quality, and depressed affect. Health Psychology, 24, 526–531.

155. Mikulincer, M., & Shaver, P. R. (2003). The attachment behavioral system in adulthood: Activation, psychodynamics,

and interpersonal processes. Advances in Experimental Social Psychology, 35, 56–152.

Troxel, W. M., Robles, T. F., Hall, M. H., & Buysse, D. J. (2007). Marital quality and the marital bed: Examining the covariation between relationship quality and sleep. Sleep Medicine, 11, 389–404.

156. Monroe, L. J. (1969). Transient changes in EEG sleep patterns of married good sleepers: The effects of altering sleeping arrangement. Psychophysiology, 6, 330–337.

157. Pankhurst, F. P., & Horne, J. A. (1994). The influence of bed partners on movement during sleep. Sleep, 17, 308–315.

158. Meadows, R., Venn, S., Hislop, J., Stanley, N., & Arber, S. (2005). Investigating couples' sleep: An evaluation of actigraphic analysis techniques. Journal of Sleep Research, 14, 377–386.

Meadows, R., Arber, S., Venn, S., Hislop, J., & Stanley, N. (2009). Exploring the interdependence of couples' rest-wake cycles: An actigraphic study. Chronobiology International, 26, 80–82.

159. Mochida, K., & Nishikawa, M. (2014). Sleep duration is affected by social relationships among sleeping partners in wild Japanese macaques. Behavioural Processes, 103, 102–104.

160. Kent de Grey, R. G., Uchino, B. N., Pietromonaco, P. R., Hogan, J. N., Smith, T. W., Cronan, S., & Trettevik, R. (2019). Strained bedfellows: An actor–partner analysis of spousal attachment insecurity and sleep quality. Annals of behavioral medicine, 53(2), 115-125.

161. Carmichael, C. L., & Reis, H. T. (2005). Attachment, sleep quality, and depressed affect. Health Psychology, 24(5), 526.

Hicks, A. M., & Diamond, L. M. (2011). Don't go to bed angry: Attachment, conflict, and affective and physiological reactivity. Personal Relationships, 18(2), 266-284.

Scharfe, E., & Eldredge, D. (2001). Associations between attachment representations and health behaviors in late adolescence. Journal of Health Psychology, 6(3), 295-307.

Sloan, E. P., Maunder, R. G., Hunter, J. J., & Moldofsky, H. (2007). Insecure attachment is associated with the α-EEG anomaly during sleep. BioPsychoSocial Medicine, 1(1), 1-6.

Troxel, W. M., Robles, T. F., Hall, M., & Buysse, D. J. (2007). Marital quality and the marital bed: Examining the covariation between relationship quality and sleep. Sleep medicine reviews, 11(5), 389-404.

Verdecias, R. N., Jean-Louis, G., Zizi, F., Casimir, G. J., & Browne, R. C. (2009). Attachment styles and sleep measures in a community-based sample of older adults. Sleep medicine, 10(6), 664-667.

162. Hasler, B. P., & Troxel, W. M. (2010). Couples' nighttime sleep efficiency and concordance: Evidence for bidirectional associations with daytime relationship functioning. Psychosomatic Medicine, 72, 794–801.

163. Smith, D. E. (1993). The standard North American family SNAF as an ideological code. Journal of Family Issues, 14, 50–65.

164. Gross, N. (2005). The detraditionalization of intimacy reconsidered. Sociological Theory, 23, 286–311

165. Burke, P. J. (1991). Identity processes and social stress. American Sociological Review, 56, 836–849.

166. McLeod, J. D. (2015). Why and how inequality matters. Journal of Health and Social Behavior, 56, 149–165.

167. Stets, J. E., & Harrod, M. M. (2004). Verification across multiple identities: The role of status. Social Psychology Quarterly, 67, 155–171.

168. Ditzen, B., Hoppmann, C. and Klumb, P. (2008) Positive Couple Interactions and Daily Cortisol: On the Stress-Protecting Role of Intimacy. Psychosomatic Medicine, 70, 883-889.

169. Paulsen, V.M. and Shaver, J.L. (1991) Stress, Support, Psychological States and Sleep. Social Science & Medicine, 32, 1237-1243.

170. Kiecolt-Glaser, J. K., & Wilson, S. J. (2017). Lovesick: How couples' relationships influence health. Annual review of clinical psychology, 13, 421-443.

171. Chen, J. H., Waite, L. J., & Lauderdale, D. S. (2015). Marriage, relationship quality, and sleep among US older adults. Journal of health and social behavior, 56(3), 356-377.

172. Chen, J. H., Waite, L. J., & Lauderdale, D. S. (2015). Marriage, relationship quality, and sleep among US older adults. Journal of health and social behavior, 56(3), 356-377.

Troxel, W. M., Buysse, D. J., Hall, M., & Matthews, K. A. (2009). Marital happiness and sleep disturbances in a multi-ethnic sample of middle-aged women. Behavioral sleep medicine, 7(1), 2-19.

173. Chen, J. H., Waite, L. J., & Lauderdale, D. S. (2015). Marriage, relationship quality, and sleep among US older adults. Journal of health and social behavior, 56(3), 356-377.
Troxel, W. M., Buysse, D. J., Hall, M., & Matthews, K. A. (2009). Marital happiness and sleep disturbances in a multi-ethnic sample of middle-aged women. Behavioral sleep medicine, 7(1), 2-19.

174. Yang, H. C., Suh, S., Kim, H., Cho, E. R., Lee, S. K., & Shin, C. (2013). Testing bidirectional relationships between marital quality and sleep disturbances: A 4-year follow-up study in a Korean cohort. Journal of psychosomatic research, 74(5), 401-406.

175. El-Sheikh, M., Kelly, R. J., Koss, K. J., & Rauer, A. J. (2015). Longitudinal relations between constructive and destructive conflict and couples' sleep. Journal of Family Psychology, 29(3), 349.

176. Hasler, B. P., & Troxel, W. M. (2010). Couples' nighttime sleep efficiency and concordance: Evidence for bidirectional associations with daytime relationship functioning. Psychosomatic medicine, 72(8), 794.

177. Hasler, B. P., & Troxel, W. M. (2010). Couples' nighttime sleep efficiency and concordance: Evidence for bidirectional associations with daytime relationship functioning. Psychosomatic medicine, 72(8), 794.

178. Gordon, A. M., & Chen, S. (2014). The role of sleep in interpersonal conflict: do sleepless nights mean worse fights? Social Psychological and Personality Science, 5(2), 168-175.

179. Kane, H. S., Slatcher, R. B., Reynolds, B. M., Repetti, R. L., & Robles, T. F. (2014). Daily self-disclosure and sleep in couples. Health Psychology, 33(8), 813.

180. McFayden, T. A., Espie, C. A., McArdle, N., Douglas, N. J., & Engleman, H. M. (2001). Controlled, prospective trial of psychosocial function before and after continuous positive airway pressure therapy. European Respiratory Journal, 18, 996–1002

181. Hasler, B. P., & Troxel, W. M. (2010). Couples' nighttime sleep efficiency and concordance: Evidence for bidirectional associations with daytime relationship functioning. Psychosomatic medicine, 72(8), 794.

182. Troxel, W. M., Braithwaite, S. R., Sandberg, J. G., & Holt-Lunstad, J. (2017). Does improving marital quality improve sleep? Results

from a marital therapy trial. Behavioral sleep medicine, 15(4), 330-343.

183. Newton, T. L., Burns, V. E., Miller, J. J., & Fernandez-Botran, G. R. (2016). Subjective sleep quality in women with divorce histories: The role of intimate partner victimization. Journal of interpersonal violence, 31(8), 1430-1452.

184. Martire, L. M., Schulz, R., Helgeson, V. S., Small, B. J., & Saghafi, E. M. (2010). Review and meta-analysis of couple-oriented interventions for chronic illness. Annals of behavioral medicine, 40(3), 325-342.

185. Song, S., Graham-Engeland, J. E., Mogle, J., & Martire, L. M. (2015). The effects of daily mood and couple interactions on the sleep quality of older adults with chronic pain. Journal of behavioral medicine, 38(6), 944-955.

186. Hasler, B. P., & Troxel, W. M. (2010). Couples' nighttime sleep efficiency and concordance: Evidence for bidirectional associations with daytime relationship functioning. Psychosomatic medicine, 72(8), 794.

187. Gordon AM, Chen S. 2014. The role of sleep in interpersonal conflict: Do sleepless nights mean worse fights? Soc. Psychol. Pers. Sci. 5:168–75

188. Dahl, R. E., & El-Sheikh, M. (2007). Considering sleep in a family context: introduction to the special issue. Journal of Family Psychology, 21(1), 1.
Troxel, W. M., Buysse, D. J., Hall, M., & Matthews, K. A. (2009). Marital happiness and sleep disturbances in a multi-ethnic sample of middle-aged women. Behavioral sleep medicine, 7(1), 2-19.

189. Nomura, K., Yamaoka, K., Nakao, M., & Yano, E. (2010). Social determinants of self-reported sleep problems in South Korea and Taiwan. Journal of psychosomatic research, 69(5), 435-440.
Troxel, W. M., Robles, T. F., Hall, M., & Buysse, D. J. (2007). Marital quality and the marital bed: Examining the covariation between relationship quality and sleep. Sleep medicine reviews, 11(5), 389-404.

190. Nordin, M., Knutsson, A., & Sundbom, E. (2008). Is disturbed sleep a mediator in the association between social support and myocardial infarction? Journal of Health Psychology, 13(1), 55-64.
Rambod, M., Ghodsbin, F., Beheshtipour, N., Raieyatpishe, A. A.,

Mohebi Noubandegani, Z., & Mohammadi-Nezhad, A. (2013). The Relationship between Perceived Social Support and Quality of Sleep in Nursing Students. Iran Journal of Nursing (2008-5923), 25(79).

Troxel, W. M., Buysse, D. J., Monk, T. H., Begley, A., & Hall, M. (2010). Does social support differentially affect sleep in older adults with versus without insomnia? Journal of Psychosomatic research, 69(5), 459-466.

191. Troxel, W. M., Buysse, D. J., Hall, M., & Matthews, K. A. (2009). Marital happiness and sleep disturbances in a multi-ethnic sample of middle-aged women. Behavioral sleep medicine, 7(1), 2-19.

192. Brummett, B. H., Babyak, M. A., Siegler, I. C., Vitaliano, P. P., Ballard, E. L., Gwyther, L. P., & Williams, R. B. (2006). Associations among perceptions of social support, negative affect, and quality of sleep in caregivers and noncaregivers. Health Psychology, 25(2), 220

193. Bolger, N., DeLongis, A., Kessler, R. C., & Schilling, E. A. (1989). Effects of daily stress on negative mood. Journal of personality and social psychology, 57(5), 808.

194. Yorgason, J. B., Godfrey, W. B., Call, V. R., Erickson, L. D., Gustafson, K. B., & Bond, A. H. (2018). Daily sleep predicting marital interactions as mediated through mood. The Journals of Gerontology: Series B, 73(3), 421-431.

195. Insana, S. P., Costello, C. R., & Montgomery-Downs, H. E. (2011). Perception of partner sleep and mood: Postpartum couples' relationship satisfaction. Journal of sex & marital therapy, 37(5), 428-440.

Strawbridge, W. J., Shema, S. J., & Roberts, R. E. (2004). Impact of spouses' sleep problems on partners. Sleep, 27(3), 527-531.

196. Troxel, W.M., Buysse, D.J., Hall, M. and Matthews, K.A. (2009) Marital Happiness and Sleep Disturbances in a Multi-Ethnic Sample of Middle-Aged Women. Behavioral Sleep Medicine, 7, 2-19.

197. Kent, R. G., Uchino, B. N., Cribbet, M. R., Bowen, K., & Smith, T. W. (2015). Social relationships and sleep quality. Annals of Behavioral Medicine, 49(6), 912-917.

198. Ailshire, J. A., & Burgard, S. A. (2012). Family relationships and troubled sleep among US adults: examining the influences of

contact frequency and relationship quality. Journal of health and social behavior, 53(2), 248-262.

199. Maranges, H. M., & McNulty, J. K. (2017). The rested relationship: Sleep benefits marital evaluations. Journal of Family Psychology, 31(1), 117.

200. Buck, A. A., & Neff, L. A. (2012). Stress spillover in early marriage: The role of self-regulatory depletion. Journal of Family Psychology, 26, 698–708.
    Vohs, K. D., Finkenauer, C., & Baumeister, R. F. (2011). The sum of friends' and lovers' self-control scores predicts relationship quality. Social Psychological and Personality Science, 2, 138–145.

201. Hagger, M. S., Wood, C., Stiff, C., & Chatzisarantis, N. L. (2010). Ego depletion and the strength model of self-control: A meta-analysis. Psychological Bulletin, 136, 495–525.

202. Wright, R. A. (2010). Sleep consistency as a mechanism for improving inhibitory system strength. Stress and Health: Journal of the International Society for the Investigation of Stress, 26, 198–199.

203. Hasler, B. P., & Troxel, W. M. (2010). Couples' nighttime sleep efficiency and concordance: Evidence for bidirectional associations with daytime relationship functioning. Psychosomatic medicine, 72(8), 794.

204. Brissette, I, & Cohen, S. (2002). The contribution of individual difference in hostility to the associations between daily interpersonal conflict, affect, and sleep. Personality and Social Psychology Bulletin, 28.
    Hoshino, K., Pasqualini, J. C., D'Oliveira, E. P., da Silva, C. P., Modesto, A. E., & Silveira, R. S. M. (2009). Is sleep deprivation involved in domestic violence? Sleep Science, 2, 14–20.

205. Keller, P. S., Blincoe, S., Gilbert, L. R., Haak, E. A., & DeWall, C. N. (2014). Sleep deprivation and dating aggression perpetration in female college students: The moderating roles of trait aggression, victimization by partner, and alcohol use. Journal of Aggression, Maltreatment & Trauma, 23(4), 351–368.

206. Rauer, A. J., & El-Sheikh, M. (2012). Reciprocal pathways between intimate partner violence and sleep in men and women. Journal of Family Psychology, 26(3), 470.

207. Kent, R. G., Uchino, B. N., Cribbet, M. R., Bowen, K., Smith, T. W.

(2015). Social relationships and sleep quality. Annals of Behavioral Medicine, 49, 912–917.

208. Hoshino, K., Pasqualini, J. C., D'Oliveira, E. P., da Silva, C. P., Modesto, A. E., & Silveira, R. S. M. (2009). Is sleep deprivation involved in domestic violence? Sleep Science, 2, 14–20.

209. Brissette, I, & Cohen, S. (2002). The contribution of individual difference in hostility to the associations between daily interpersonal conflict, affect, and sleep. Personality and Social Psychology Bulletin, 28.

210. Keller, P. S., Blincoe, S., Gilbert, L. R., Haak, E. A., & DeWall, C. N. (2014). Sleep deprivation and dating aggression perpetration in female college students: The moderating roles of trait aggression, victimization by partner, and alcohol use. Journal of Aggression, Maltreatment & Trauma, 23(4), 351–368.

211. Rauer, A. J., & El-Sheikh, M. (2012). Reciprocal pathways between intimate partner violence and sleep in men and women. Journal of Family Psychology, 26(3), 470.

212. Yoo, S., Gujar, N, Hu, P., Jolesz, F. A., & Walker, M. P. (2007). The human emotional brain without sleep: A prefrontal amygdala disconnect. Current Biology, 17, R877–R878.

213. Carstensen, L. L., Gottman, J. M., & Levenson, R. W. (1995). Emotional behavior in long-term marriage. Psychology and Aging, 10(1), 140.

214. Keller, P. S., Haak, E. A., DeWall, C. N., & Renzetti, C. (2019). Poor sleep is associated with greater marital aggression: The role of self control. Behavioral sleep medicine, 17(2), 174-180.

215. Dahl, R. E. (1996). The regulation of sleep and arousal: Development and psychopathology. Development and Psychopathology, 8(1), 3–27.

216. Rauer, A. J., Kelly, R. J., Buckhalt, J. A., & El-Sheikh, M. (2010). Sleeping with one eye open: Marital abuse as an antecedent of poor sleep. Journal of Family Psychology, 24(6), 667.

217. Rauer, A. J., Kelly, R. J., Buckhalt, J. A., & El-Sheikh, M. (2010). Sleeping with one eye open: Marital abuse as an antecedent of poor sleep. Journal of Family Psychology, 24(6), 667.

218. Yoo, S.-S., Gujar, N., Hu, P., Jolesz, F. A., & Walker, M. P. (2007). The human emotional brain without sleep: A prefrontalamygdala disconnect. Current Biology, 17, 7723–7728

219. Selvi, Y., Gulec, M., Agargun, M. Y., & Besiroglu, L. (2007). Mood changes after sleep deprivation in morningness–eveningness chronotypes in healthy individuals. Journal of Sleep Research, 16, 241–244.

Zohar, D., Tzischinsky, O., Epstein, R., & Lavie, P. (2005). The effects of sleep loss on medical residents' emotional reactions to work events: A cognitive-energy model. Journal of Sleep and Sleep Disorders Research, 28, 47–54

220. Killgore, W. D. S., Kahn-Greene, E. T., Lipizzi, E. L., Newman, R. A., Kamimori, G. H., & Balkin, T. J. (2008). Sleep deprivation reduces perceived emotional intelligence and constructive thinking skills. Sleep Medicine, 9, 517–526.

van der Helm, E., Gujar, N., & Walker, M. P. (2010). Sleep deprivation impairs the accurate recognition of human emotions. Sleep, 33, 335–342

221. Bissonette, V. L., Rusbult, C. E., & Kilpatrick, S. D. (1997). Empathic accuracy and marital conflict resolution. In W. Ickes (Ed.), Empathic accuracy (pp. 251–281). New York, NY: The Guilford Press.

Fruzzetti, A. E., & Iverson, K. A. (2006). Intervening with couples and families to treat emotion dysregulation and psychopathology. In D. K. Snyder, J. Simpson, & J. N. Hughes (Eds.), Emotion regulation in couples and families: Pathways to dysfunction and health. Washington, DC: American Psychological Association.

222. Harrison, Y., & Horne, J. A. (2000). The impact of sleep deprivation on decision-making: A review. Journal of Experimental Psychology: Applied, 6, 236–249.

Linde, L., & Bergström, M. (1992). The effect of one night without sleep on problem-solving and immediate recall. Psychological Research, 54, 127–136.

223. Keller, P. S., Haak, E. A., DeWall, C. N., & Renzetti, C. (2019). Poor sleep is associated with greater marital aggression: The role of self control. Behavioral sleep medicine, 17(2), 174-180.

224. Schlarb, A. A., Claßen, M., Schuster, E. S., Neuner, F., & Hautzinger, M. (2015). Did you sleep well, darling? – link between sleep quality and relationship quality. Health, 7(12), 1747.

225. El-Sheikh, M., Kelly, R. and Rauer, A. (2013) Quick to Berate, Slow to Sleep: Interpartner Psychological Conflict, Mental Health, and Sleep. Health Psychology, 32, 1057-1066.

Rauer, A.J., Kelly, R.J., Buckhalt, J.A. and El-Sheikh, M. (2010) Sleeping with One Eye Open: Marital Abuse as an Antecedent of Poor Sleep. Journal of Family Psychology, 24, 667-677.

Rauer, A.J. and El-Sheikh, M. (2012) Reciprocal Pathways between Intimate Partner Violence and Sleep in Men and Women. Journal of Family Psychology, 26, 470-477. http://dx.doi.org/10.1037/a0027828

226. Gordon, A.M. and Chen, S. (2014) The Role of Sleep in Interpersonal Conflict: Do Sleepless Nights Mean Worse Fights? Social Psychological and Personality Science, 5, 168-175.

227. Birditt, K. S., Brown, E., Orbuch, T. L., & McIlvane, J. M. (2010). Marital conflict behaviors and implications for divorce over 16 years. Journal of Marriage and Family, 72(5), 1188-1204.

228. Walters, E. M., Phillips, A. J., Hamill, K., Norton, P. J., & Drummond, S. P. (2020). Anxiety predicts dyadic sleep characteristics in couples experiencing insomnia but not in couples without sleep disorders. Journal of Affective Disorders, 273, 122-130.

229. Revenson, T. A., Marín-Chollom, A. M., Rundle, A. G., Wisnivesky, J., & Neugut, A. I. (2016). Hey Mr. Sandman: dyadic effects of anxiety, depressive symptoms and sleep among married couples. Journal of behavioral medicine, 39(2), 225-232.

230. Uchino, B. N., Scott, E., de Grey, R. G. K., Hogan, J., Trettevik, R., Cronan, S., ... & Bosch, J. A. (2019). Sleep quality and inflammation in married heterosexual couples: an actor-partner analysis. International journal of behavioral medicine, 26(3), 247-254.

231. Wilson, S. J., Jaremka, L. M., Fagundes, C. P., Andridge, R., Peng, J., Malarkey, W. B., & Kiecolt-Glaser, J. K. (2017). Shortened sleep fuels inflammatory responses to marital conflict: Emotion regulation matters. Psychoneuroendocrinology, 79, 74-83.

232. Shih, Y. C., Han, S. H., & Burr, J. A. (2019). Are spouses' sleep problems a mechanism through which health is compromised? Evidence regarding insomnia and heart disease. Annals of Behavioral Medicine, 53(4), 345-357.

233. Walters, E. M., Phillips, A. J., Boardman, J. M., Norton, P. J., & Drummond, S. P. (2020). Vulnerability and resistance to sleep disruption by a partner: A study of bed-sharing couples. Sleep health, 6(4), 506-512.

234. Gunn, H. E., Buysse, D. J., Hasler, B. P., Begley, A., & Troxel,

W. M. (2015). Sleep concordance in couples is associated with relationship characteristics. Sleep, 38(6), 933-939.

Dittami, J., Keckeis, M., Machatschke, I., Katina, S., Zeitlhofer, J., & Kloesch, G. (2007). Sex differences in the reactions to sleeping in pairs versus sleeping alone in humans. Sleep and Biological Rhythms, 5(4), 271-276.

Troxel, W. M. (2010). It's more than sex: Exploring the dyadic nature of sleep and implications for health. Psychosomatic medicine, 72(6), 578.

Pankhurst, F. P., & Home, J. A. (1994). The influence of bed partners on movement during sleep. Sleep, 17(4), 308-315.

235. Gunn, H. E., Buysse, D. J., Matthews, K. A., Kline, C. E., Cribbet, M. R., & Troxel, W. M. (2017). Sleep–wake concordance in couples is inversely associated with cardiovascular disease risk markers. Sleep, 40(1), zsw028.

Uchino, B. N., Scott, E., de Grey, R. G. K., Hogan, J., Trettevik, R., Cronan, S., ... & Bosch, J. A. (2019). Sleep quality and inflammation in married heterosexual couples: an actor-partner analysis. International journal of behavioral medicine, 26(3), 247-254.

Strawbridge, W. J., Shema, S. J., & Roberts, R. E. (2004). Impact of spouses' sleep problems on partners. Sleep, 27(3), 527-531.

Revenson, T. A., Marín-Chollom, A. M., Rundle, A. G., Wisnivesky, J., & Neugut, A. I. (2016). Hey Mr. Sandman: dyadic effects of anxiety, depressive symptoms and sleep among married couples. Journal of behavioral medicine, 39(2), 225-232.

236. Saxbe, D., & Repetti, R. L. (2010). For better or worse? Coregulation of couples' cortisol levels and mood states. Journal of personality and social psychology, 98(1), 92.

Timmons, A. C., Margolin, G., & Saxbe, D. E. (2015). Physiological linkage in couples and its implications for individual and interpersonal functioning: A literature review. Journal of Family Psychology, 29(5), 720.

237. Gunn, H. E., Buysse, D. J., Hasler, B. P., Begley, A., & Troxel, W. M. (2015). Sleep concordance in couples is associated with relationship characteristics. Sleep, 38(6), 933-939.

Pankhurst, F. P., & Home, J. A. (1994). The influence of bed partners on movement during sleep. Sleep, 17(4), 308-315.

Gunn, H. E., Buysse, D. J., Matthews, K. A., Kline, C. E., Cribbet,

M. R., & Troxel, W. M. (2017). Sleep–wake concordance in couples is inversely associated with cardiovascular disease risk markers. Sleep, 40(1), zsw028.

Hasler, B. P., & Troxel, W. M. (2010). Couples' nighttime sleep efficiency and concordance: Evidence for bidirectional associations with daytime relationship functioning. Psychosomatic medicine, 72(8), 794.

Meadows, R., Venn, S., Hislop, J., Stanley, N., & Arber, S. (2005). Investigating couples' sleep: an evaluation of actigraphic analysis techniques. Journal of Sleep Research, 14(4), 377-386.

238. Gunn, H. E., Buysse, D. J., Hasler, B. P., Begley, A., & Troxel, W. M. (2015). Sleep concordance in couples is associated with relationship characteristics. Sleep, 38(6), 933-939.

239. Pankhurst, F. P., & Home, J. A. (1994). The influence of bed partners on movement during sleep. Sleep, 17(4), 308-315.

240. Gunn, H. E., Buysse, D. J., Hasler, B. P., Begley, A., & Troxel, W. M. (2015). Sleep concordance in couples is associated with relationship characteristics. Sleep, 38(6), 933-939.

Pankhurst, F. P., & Home, J. A. (1994). The influence of bed partners on movement during sleep. Sleep, 17(4), 308-315.

241. Dittami, J., Keckeis, M., Machatschke, I., Katina, S., Zeitlhofer, J., & Kloesch, G. (2007). Sex differences in the reactions to sleeping in pairs versus sleeping alone in humans. Sleep and Biological Rhythms, 5(4), 271-276.

Meadows, R., Venn, S., Hislop, J., Stanley, N., & Arber, S. (2005). Investigating couples' sleep: an evaluation of actigraphic analysis techniques. Journal of Sleep Research, 14(4), 377-386.

Spiegelhalder, K., Regen, W., Siemon, F., Kyle, S. D., Baglioni, C., Feige, B., ... & Riemann, D. (2017). Your place or mine? Does the sleep location matter in young couples? Behavioral sleep medicine, 15(2), 87-96.

242. Dittami, J., Keckeis, M., Machatschke, I., Katina, S., Zeitlhofer, J., & Kloesch, G. (2007). Sex differences in the reactions to sleeping in pairs versus sleeping alone in humans. Sleep and Biological Rhythms, 5(4), 271-276.

243. Spiegelhalder, K., Regen, W., Siemon, F., Kyle, S. D., Baglioni, C., Feige, B., ... & Riemann, D. (2017). Your place or mine? Does the sleep location matter in young couples? Behavioral sleep

medicine, 15(2), 87-96.

244. Gunn, H. E., Buysse, D. J., Matthews, K. A., Kline, C. E., Cribbet, M. R., & Troxel, W. M. (2016). Sleep-wake concordance in couples is inversely associated with cardiovascular disease risk markers. Sleep, 40, 1–10.

245. Troxel, W. M. (2010). It's more than sex: Exploring the dyadic nature of sleep and implications for health. Psychosomatic medicine, 72(6), 578.

246. Richter, K., Adam, S., Geiss, L., Peter, L., & Niklewski, G. (2016). Two in a bed: The influence of couple sleeping and chronotypes on relationship and sleep. An overview. Chronobiology International, 33, 1464– 1472.

247. Peter Hauri The sleep disorders, Upjohn, 1977

248. https://wellcomecollection.org/works/hpj9ntza/items?canvas=1& langCode=eng&sierraId=b21694862

249. https://play.google.com/store/books/details?id=ewAAAAAAQAAJ &rdid=book-ewAAAAAAQAAJ&rdot=1

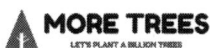